Fundamentals of Color:
Shade Matching and Communication in Esthetic De

Fundamentals of COLOR

Shade Matching and Communication in Esthetic Dentistry

Stephen J. Chu, DMD, MSD, CDT, MDT
Director, Advanced and International CDE Programs in Aesthetic Dentistry
Clinical Associate Professor
Department of Implant Dentistry
Division of Reconstructive and Prosthodontic Sciences
New York University College of Dentistry
New York, New York

Alessandro Devigus, Dr med dent
Private Practice
Bülach, Switzerland

Adam J. Mieleszko, CDT
Ceramist
New York, New York

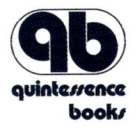

Quintessence Publishing Co, Inc
Chicago, Berlin, Tokyo, Copenhagen, London, Paris, Milan, Barcelona, Istanbul, São Paulo, New Delhi, Moscow, Prague, and Warsaw

For my daughters, Melissa and Stephanie, and my teacher, Dr Ralph A. Yuodelis.
—SJC

For my family, Beatrice, Raffael, and Valentin.
—AD

For Iga Jarnutowska and in memory of Borys Mieleszko.
—AJM

Library of Congress Cataloguing in Publication Data

Chu, Stephen J.
  Fundamentals of color : shade matching and communication in esthetic dentistry / Stephen J. Chu, Alessandro Devigus, Adam Mieleszko.
      p. ; cm.
  Includes bibliographical references and index.
  ISBN 0-86715-434-9 (pbk.)
  1. Dentistry—Aesthetic aspects. 2. Color in dentistry. 3. Dental materials. 4. Dental ceramics.
  [DNLM: 1. Esthetics, Dental. 2. Dental Prosthesis Design. 3. Prosthesis Coloring. WU 100 C559f 2004] I. Devigus, Alessandro. II. Mieleszko, Adam. III. Title.

RK54.C48 2004
617.6'95—dc22

2004006061

©2004 Quintessence Publishing Co, Inc

Quintessence Publishing Co, Inc
551 Kimberly Drive
Carol Stream, IL 60188
www.quintpub.com

Photos on pages 77 and 101 courtesy of Irfan Ahmad, BDS, Middlesex, UK.

All rights reserved. This book or any part thereof may not be reproduced, stored in a retrieval system, or transmitted in any form or by any means, electronic, mechanical, photocopying, or otherwise, without prior written permission of the publisher.

Editor: Kathryn O'Malley
Production and Design: Dawn Hartman

Printed in China

Table of Contents

Foreword   vii

Preface   ix

1 Color Theory   1
The Physics of Color
Color Reproduction
Color in Dentistry

2 Elements Affecting Color   19
Illumination
Contrast Effects
Viewer-Associated Effects
Restorative Materials Selection

3 Conventional Shade Matching   51
Step-by-Step Process
Shade Guide Systems
Recommended Protocol
Special Considerations for Direct Composites

4 Technology-Based Shade Matching 77

Development of Technological Shade Systems
Measurement Systems
Types of Technological Shade Systems
Step-by-Step Process
Recommended Protocol

5 Recommended Shade-Matching Protocol 101

Seven Steps to a Successful Shade Match

Appendix: Clinical Cases 117

Single Anterior All-Ceramic (Procera) Crown
Single Anterior All-Ceramic (In-Ceram) Crown
Single Anterior Implant-Supported Metal-Ceramic Crown
Single Anterior Ceramic Laminate Veneer
Two Anterior All-Ceramic Crowns
Two Anterior All-Ceramic Crowns with One Anterior Metal-Ceramic Crown
Four Anterior Ceramic Laminate Veneers
Single Posterior All-Ceramic Crown
Ten Ceramic Laminate Veneers to Match Bleached Teeth
Two Anterior Direct Composite Restorations

Index 155

Foreword

In the span of my dental career, dentistry has made spectacular improvements in mimicking the natural colors of teeth with restorative materials. In the early 1960s, metal ceramics presented exciting new possibilities for tooth colors, as well as soft tissue response, longevity, and esthetics. In general, clinicians have had little understanding about color, and even less has been taught. Several contemporary clinicians contributed enormously to our knowledge of the art and science of color. There was Bruce Clark in the 1930s and then Robert C. Sproull, Jack D. Preston, and Stephen F. Bergen in the 1970s.

John W. McLean, a giant in the dental profession, introduced us to high-strength all-porcelain restorations with aluminous porcelain in 1965. The bar was raised for color in dental porcelain. Artistic laboratory technicians made immense progress with internal colors and the management of opacity and translucency. By the 1990s, adhesive dentistry, composites, and myriad all-ceramic materials gave us the artistic capacity to reproduce the colors and light response of natural teeth.

The authors of this text, Stephen J. Chu, Alessandro Devigus, and Adam J. Mieleszko, have made an outstanding contribution to the practice and theory of color management in contemporary dentistry. Updating is a way of life, and the flood of new materials and techniques makes this text all the more valuable to students, general practitioners, and specialists. A concise introduction to color theory and how it applies to dentistry is followed by important information about elements affecting color to aid the clinician and technician with problem solving. Special attention has been given to shade matching with a step-by-step protocol. Direct composites and layering techniques receive careful consideration. In particular, the chapter on digitized shade-matching technology provides the reader with valuable insight into color measurement technology and its applications for laboratories and patients. Finally, an extensive presentation of clinical cases from single anterior crowns and composites to multiple anterior restorations is used to illustrate the full extent of the text.

It should be noted that the science of color in dentistry always requires skill by the user. In particular, there is a lack of standards in the production of dental ceramic frits. The variables of hue, value, chroma, and translucency from batch to batch and between companies require unusual artistic skills from ceramists to produce prescriptive shades. Perfect shade measurement will not produce comparable shade matching unless realistic standards are established by manufacturers. In the meantime, we need to be especially empathetic to dental laboratories until the science and art of color in dentistry come together.

The authors have produced a text on shade matching and communication that fulfills a genuine need. I found it to be a refreshing approach to color and am especially privileged to write this foreword.

Lloyd L. Miller, DMD
Clinical Professor
Graduate and Postgraduate Prosthodontics
Tufts University School of Dental Medicine
Boston, Massachusetts

Preface

The study of color is an integral part of esthetic dentistry. If the color of a restoration is off—even slightly—the mistake can be glaringly evident; it looks fake, and the patient is unhappy. Obviously, this is an undesirable result.

Unfortunately, color is also tricky. Slight variances in shade play with our eyes, our minds, and, ultimately, our dentistry. The illumination in the dental treatment room, optical illusions, color blindness, nutrition, and fatigue are among the dental professional's ongoing obstacles to successful shade matching. It is necessary to understand these challenges and the basic mechanisms of color in order to achieve consistent esthetic shade results. However, most of the dental literature on color theory does not improve the reader's understanding; rather, it further compounds the complexity. Moreover, color education seems to be absent within the dental school curriculum. What is needed is a resource that distills all the data and breaks down the abstract science of color into the essential details. This text was written to simplify the study of color and help readers quantify and communicate shade easily and accurately.

Fundamentals of Color first explains the basics of color theory, then illuminates the factors that can affect the perception of color. Next, the recommended protocol for conventional and technology-based shade matching are detailed separately. Finally, an approach combining both methods is outlined in chapter 5, providing the reader with a technique that almost ensures an accurate shade match the first time, every time. Throughout the text, there are hints and tips to enhance the reader's comprehension and clinical results. Also included is an appendix describing clinical cases in which the recommended protocol was followed to achieve esthetic and predictable results.

This book is intended for anyone seeking to gain a better understanding of the complexities of shade matching, advance their esthetic dentistry skills, and increase the natural quality of their restorative work. Although we are all health care providers first, we are also artists. With a good working knowledge of color, your artistry will become as *natural* as your dentistry.

Without the support, dedication, and passion of many people, this book would not have been possible.

First, we would like to thank the people at X-Rite, Inc: Mike Ferrara, Tom Nyenhuis, Kevin Aamodt, Jim Overbeck, and Shannon Gary, who greatly contributed to our knowledge in the field of color science. We would also like to recognize Dustin Ewing from MHT Optic Research for explaining the use of the SpectroShade system. Thanks to Dr William Devisio and Bernal Stewart from Colgate-Palmolive Co for the present and future collaborative clinical research projects in the area of vital bleaching. To the Heraeus-Kulzer-Jelenko Co, especially Gerrit Steen, Chris Holden, Dr Mark Pitel, and Dennis Fraioli, thank you for providing the beautiful synthetic ceramic material used in the case restorations. We would also like to recognize Steve Wright, from Lanmark Group, who helped distill our thoughts and ideas in the writing of this body of knowledge. Special thanks to the staff of Quintessence Publishing Co, who made this book into a reality.

We would also like to thank Dr Irfan Ahmad, whose contributions not only to this book but also to the specialties of fixed prosthodontics, esthetic dentistry, and dental photography have been an inspiration to practitioners globally. We are indebted to Dr Didier Dietschi, whose research in direct restorative composite materials has set the standard in resin composite color science, and his colleagues, Dr Stephano Ardu and Ivo Krejci, for the direct restorative case report they contributed to this book. Our appreciation also goes to Drs Stefan Paul and Ed McLaren, whose previous and ongoing studies in the field of technology-based color systems have considerably increased our knowledge base. We would also like to thank Giordano Lombardi, CDT, whose technical skills, techniques, and working relationship have solidified the highest standard of excellence in the area of esthetic restorative dentistry in Switzerland.

Special thanks to Dr Galip Gürel (Istanbul, Turkey), whose textbook on ceramic laminate veneers opened our eyes to the world of cosmetic restorative dentistry and color. Thanks also to Assistant Dean Kendall Beachman and Dr Dennis Tarnow at New York University College of Dentistry for their motivation and inspiration. Finally, our appreciation goes to Jason Kim, CDT, for imparting his knowledge and skill in the fields of color and translucency.

1 COLOR THEORY

In this chapter:
- The physics of color
- Color reproduction
- Color in dentistry

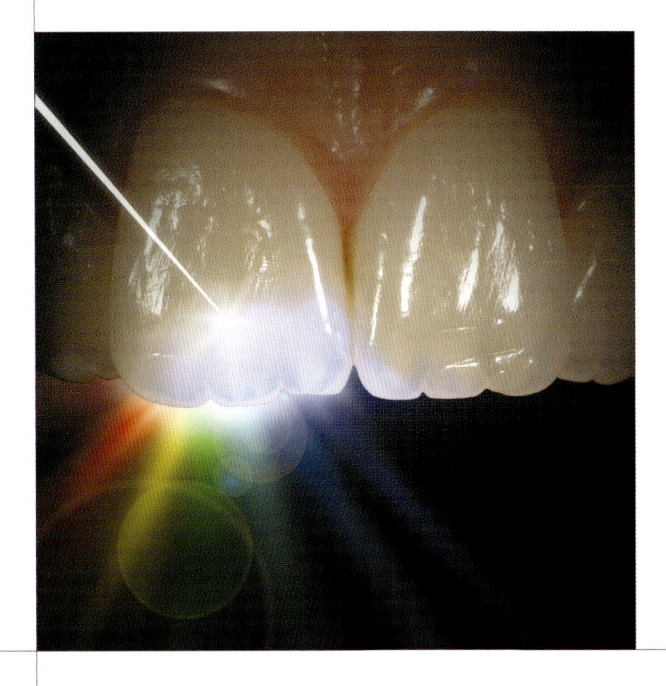

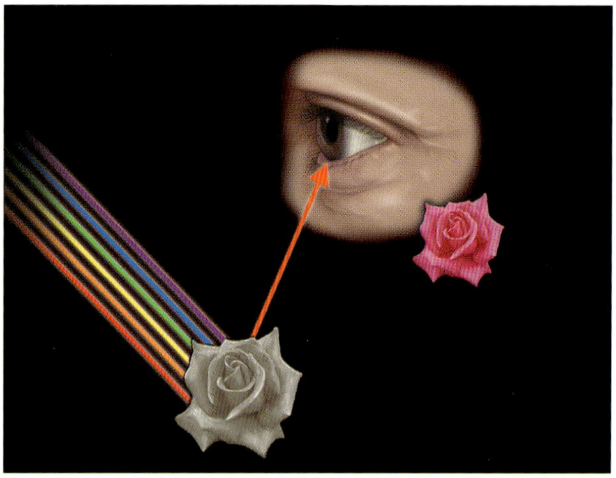

1 Color Theory

Fig 1-1
The wavelengths of light reflect off the object (a rose), resulting in the perception of color (pink) by the viewer.

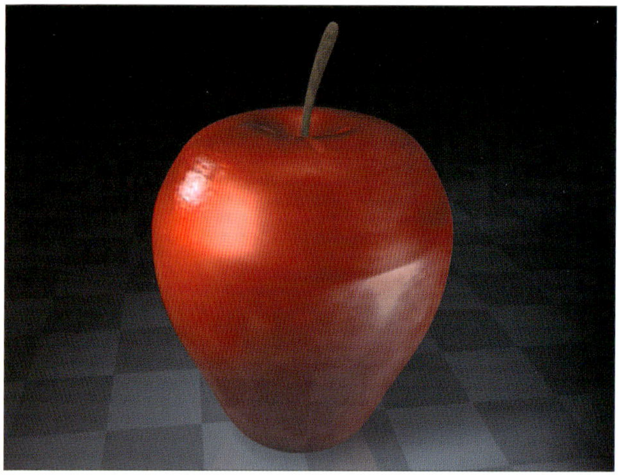

Fig 1-2
A red apple. Its specific color description is subjective and debatable, stemming from an emotional or visceral response.

Many have long pondered the question: If a tree falls in the woods and there is no one there to hear it, does it make a sound? In color theory the question becomes: If the petals of a rose are pink and there is no one there to view them, are they actually pink? According to color theorists, the answer is *no*. The reason for this surprising answer is that in order for a color to exist, there needs to be an interaction between three elements: light, an object, and a viewer (Fig 1-1). If all three elements are not present, color as we know it does not exist.

Color is best described as an *abstract science*. Color appeals to the visceral and emotional senses. Color is personal; each individual will view the same object differently. Take, for example, the apple shown in Fig 1-2. Most would define its color as *red*; others might take it a step further and describe it as *cranberry red* or *vibrant ruby red*. It is often difficult to come to a consensus based on visual assessment alone. There are numerous factors that influence an individual's color perception, including lighting conditions, background effects, color blindness, binocular differences, eye fatigue, age, and other physiologic factors (see chapter 2). But even in the absence of these physical considerations, each observer will interpret color differently based on his or her past experiences with color and resulting color references. Each individual also verbally defines an object's color differently.[1-9]

However, there are quantifiable aspects of color that are important for the dental practitioner to understand. Basic knowledge of how color is perceived and reproduced will aid the clinician in evaluating and matching shades in the dental practice.

The Physics of Color

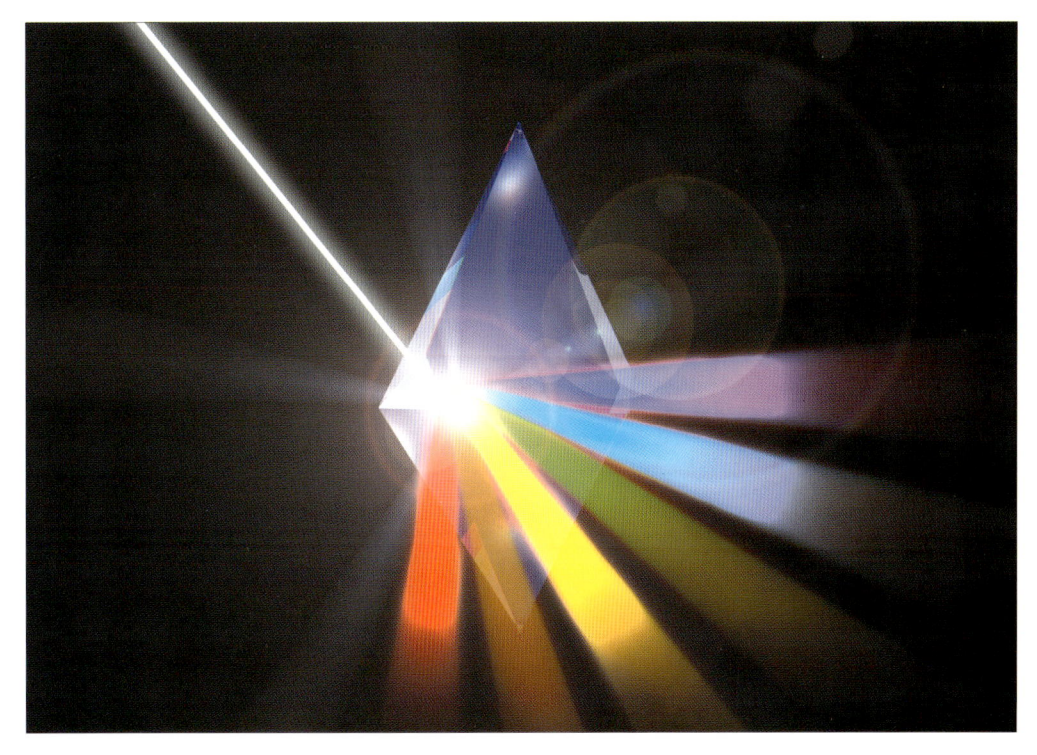

Fig 1-3
Dispersion of light through a prism breaks the light up into its component colored frequencies, which are called *wavelengths*.

The Physics of Color

Although color is generally perceived as an art form, there is a true science behind color theory. Isaac Newton was the first to break down the physics of color. He found that a beam of white light could be separated into component colors, or *wavelengths*, by passing it through a prism (Fig 1-3). Newton described the resulting continuous series of colors as a *spectrum*, and named these colors in the following order: red, orange, yellow, green, blue, indigo, and violet, as represented by the commonly used mnemonic association Roy G. Biv. These wavelengths are perceived by the three types of color receptors (called *cones*) in the human eye as variations of red, green, and blue light. The human eye can perceive only these wavelengths of light, hence the term *visible light spectrum*. In physical terms, the wavelengths of visible light range from approximately 400 to 700 nm (Figs 1-4 and 1-5). Each hue is accurately defined by its wavelength or frequency[1] (Table 1-1).

1 Color Theory

Fig 1-4
The wavelengths of visible light range from 400 nm (violet) to 700 nm (red).

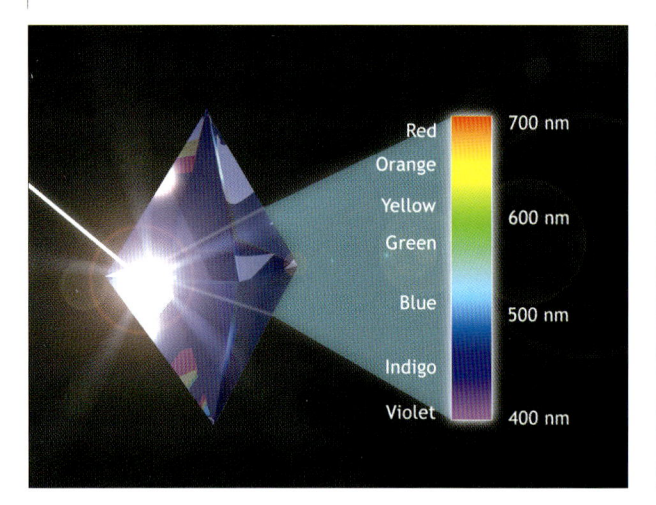

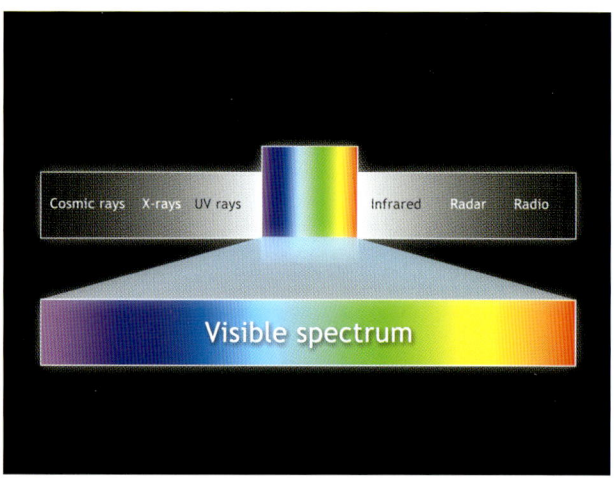

Fig 1-5
The visible light spectrum relative to the whole electromagnetic spectrum.

TABLE 1-1 WAVELENGTHS OF COLORS

Color	Wavelength (nm)*
Red	650–800
Orange	590–649
Yellow	550–589
Green	490–539
Blue	460–489
Indigo	440–459
Violet	390–439

*1 nm = 0.000001 mm.

Newton's significant breakthrough in the study of color science shifted attention to the light source.[10] His observation was simple: White light contains all colors. If an object appears to be a particular color, this means that the light reaching our eyes when viewing that object has somehow been changed by the object. In other words, it is the interaction of the light with the object that allows perception of color. Therefore, without light, there would be no color.

The basic process of color perception can be described as follows. Light is *emitted* from a light source. This light may reach the eye directly, or it may either strike or pass through an object. If the light interacts with an object, some of the light is *absorbed* by the object. The wavelengths that are not

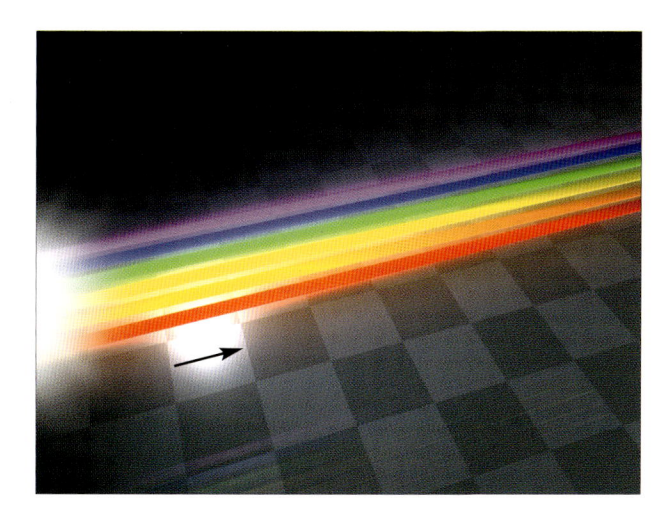

Fig 1-6
Emission of light.

absorbed (ie, those that are reflected, transmitted, or emitted directly to the eye) are perceived by receptor cells (ie, rods and cones) in the eye and recognized by the brain as a specific color. The individual components of this process are described in more detail below.

Emission

Emission of light from a source occurs through a chemical or physical process (Fig 1-6). Every process releases more light at certain wavelengths than at others. To create perfectly white light, a light source would have to emit exactly the same amount of each wavelength. In some cases, emissive objects are intended to produce specific colors. These objects, such as computer monitors, produce color by emitting light with distinct wavelength compositions of red, green, and blue light. This process is discussed in greater detail later in this chapter.

No light source can emit perfectly white light, ie, exactly the same amount of each wavelength. This affects color perception since there are only certain wavelengths (colors) being produced to interact with an object, which explains why the same object will appear to be different colors when viewed using different light sources (see chapter 2).

1 Color Theory

Fig 1-7
Transmission of light.

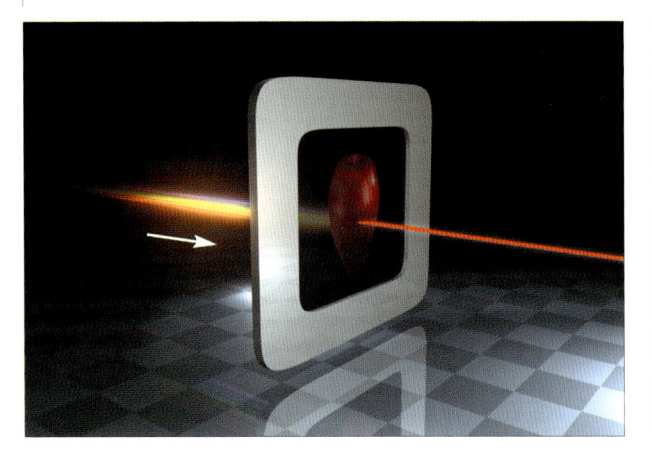

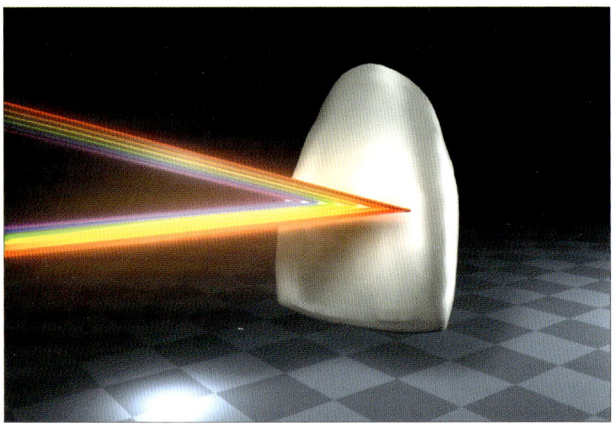

Fig 1-8
Reflection of light.

Transmission and absorption

Transmission occurs when light passes through a transparent or translucent material, such as a slide or film (Fig 1-7). If light encounters molecules or larger particles in the material, some wavelengths of light will be *absorbed*. The number of light rays and the specific wavelengths (colors) that are absorbed are determined by the density and makeup of the material the light travels through; the wavelengths that are transmitted (referred to as *spectral data*) compose the color that is perceived. If the material is completely transparent, all light is transmitted, and the color white is perceived. If the material is completely opaque, all light is absorbed, and the color black is perceived. In most cases, however, some of the wavelengths (colors) are absorbed and others transmitted. If this occurs, the color that is perceived corresponds to the wavelengths that are transmitted. For example, if a material absorbs red wavelengths and transmits green and blue wavelengths, a combination of green and blue (referred to as *cyan*) is perceived.

Reflection and absorption

Reflection occurs when light rays strike a solid object, such as an apple or a photograph, and then bounce off of it (Fig 1-8). Depending on the molecular structure or density of the object or medium, certain wavelengths (colors) may be *absorbed*

The Physics of Color

Fig 1-9
Diagram showing the percentage of light wavelengths that are reflected by an object. The percentage is measured every 10 nm along the visible light spectrum (400 to 700 nm). The resulting pattern is called a *spectral curve* and is analogous to the color fingerprint of an object.

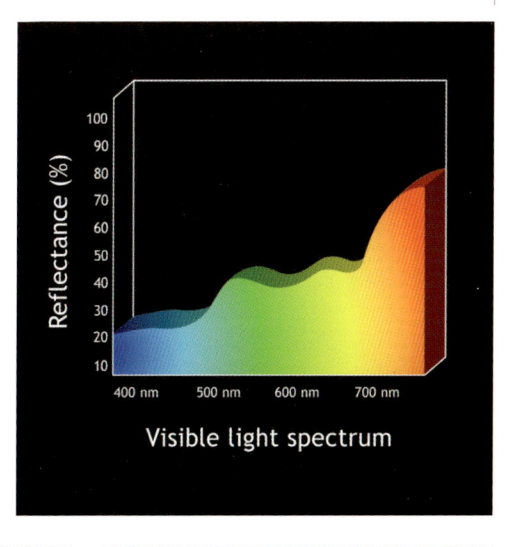

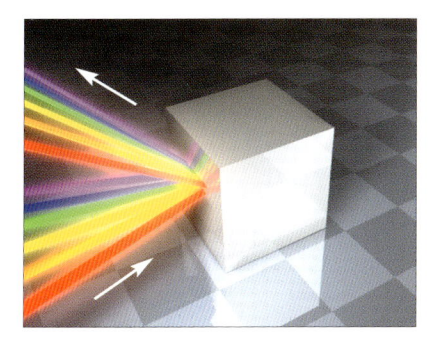

Fig 1-10
A perfectly white object would reflect all wavelengths of light.

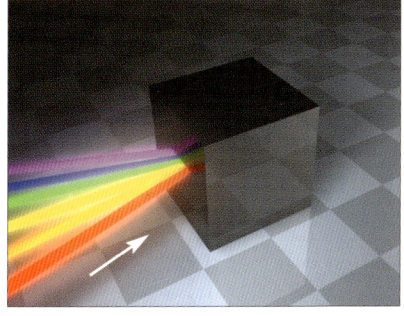

Fig 1-11
A perfectly black object would absorb all wavelengths of light.

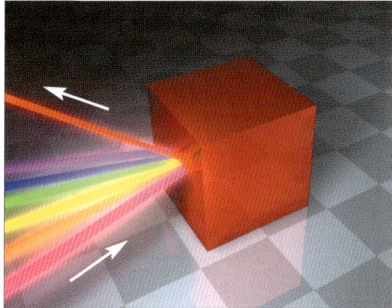

Fig 1-12
A red object reflects red light and absorbs all other wavelengths.

rather than reflected. The wavelengths that are reflected compose the color that is perceived (Fig 1-9). Theoretically, an object that reflects all light would be perceived as white (Fig 1-10), and an object that absorbs all light would be perceived as black (Fig 1-11). In most cases, however, the object absorbs some wavelengths (colors) and reflects others (Fig 1-12). If this occurs, the object is perceived to be the color of the wavelengths that are reflected. For example, an object that absorbs green wavelengths but reflects red and blue wavelengths is perceived as a combination of red and blue (referred to as *magenta*).

The surface properties of the object can affect the reflection, transmission, and absorption of light. Outside conditions such as the lighting and variability of the human eye have no effect on an object's spectral data.

Color Theory

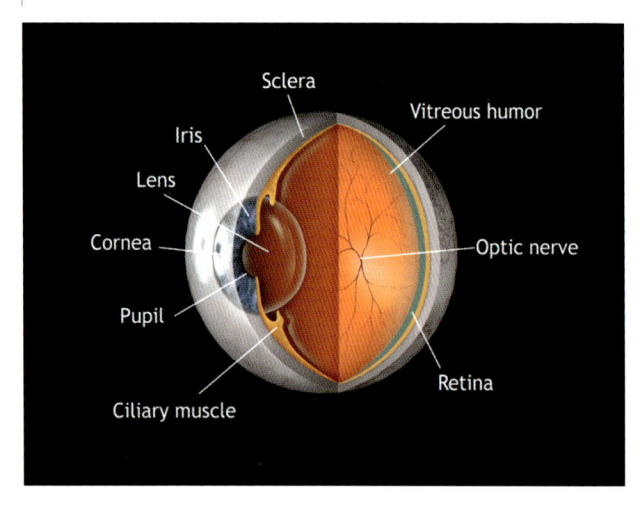

Fig 1-13
The retina of the eye contains three types of cone cells responsible for color perception, as well as rod cells, which are responsible for perception of lightness and darkness.

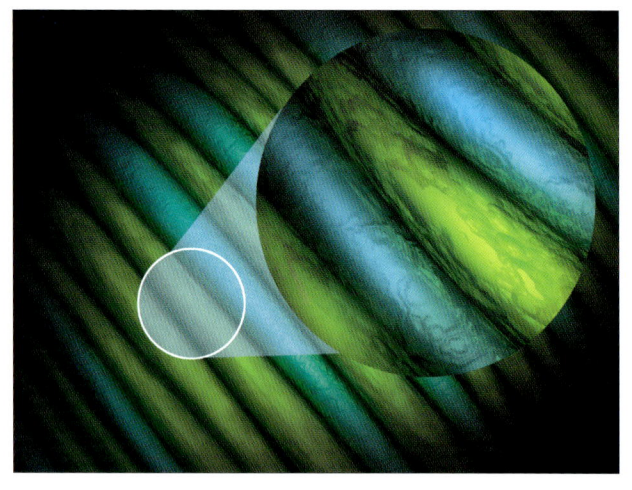

Fig 1-14
There are less cone cells *(aqua)* in the retina than there are rod cells *(green)*.

Perception

The wavelengths that reach the eye, whether by emission, transmission, or reflection, are received by the sensory cells on the retina called the *rods* and *cones* (Figs 1-13 and 1-14). The rods perceive the brightness of the color, ie, the intensity of the light rays reaching the eye. The cones perceive the *hue*, ie, the color. As discussed previously, the human eye contains three different types of cones, each one responsive to wavelengths approximating the colors red, green, and blue, respectively. Variations of these wavelengths will stimulate each cone at different intensities. The cone cells then send signals to the brain, which translates the signals into colors (Fig 1-15).

The key point to understand is that the wavelength pattern that is perceived by the eye is the color's fingerprint.[1] This fingerprint is formulated from spectral data gathered from the wavelengths of light reflected from an object. It is plotted, in reference to percentage of reflectance and wavelength interval distribution, as a spectral reflectance curve (see Fig 1-9). Therefore, in Fig 1-2, the apple itself is not red; the color that is perceived is only in the form of reflected wavelengths, and the color we sense and remember as red really exists only in our minds (Table 1-2).

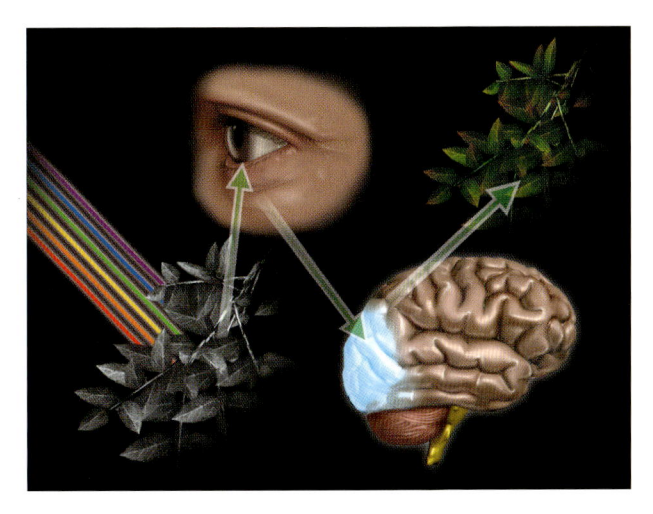

Fig 1-15
Color perception occurs in the brain.

TABLE 1-2 PSYCHOPHYSIOLOGIC REALITIES OF COLOR PERCEPTION

Mode of perception	Psychophysiologic reality
Physical	Wavelength of light
Psychophysical	Reception of light wavelength by the eye
Psychologic	Interpretation of light wavelength by the brain

Color Reproduction

Color is reproduced by means of three-dimensional color models that are based on the same mechanism by which color is perceived by the human eye (referred to as *tristimulus data*) as well as the emission, reflection, or transmission of light, depending on the medium. Colors may appear to be different depending on how they are reproduced.

Tristimulus data: Properties that describe how the color of the object appears to the observer or how the color data would be reproduced on a device such as a computer monitor or printer in terms of coordinates/values.

1 Color Theory

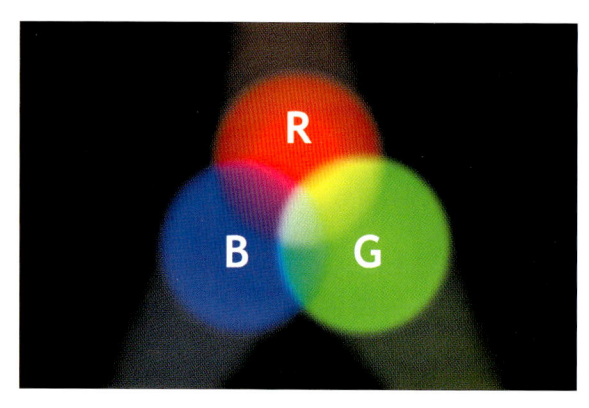

Fig 1-16
When red, green, and blue wavelengths are mixed together, white light is created.

Emissive media: RGB color model

Electronic media such as computer monitors and television sets create color by emitting wavelengths that are mixtures of red, green, and blue (RGB) light to stimulate the cones in the human eye. Such media therefore can produce a color spectrum that includes nearly all of the colors in the visible spectrum. Theoretically, if the RGB wavelengths were to be combined, white light would result (Fig 1-16). For this reason, red, green, and blue are referred to as the *additive primary colors*: From black, color is created by *adding* certain amounts of RGB wavelengths of light.

The process by which images are captured to be reproduced on emissive media (eg, the capture of images by a digital camera) is similar to the process that occurs when the human eye perceives color. A digital camera picks up tiny pixels of red, green, and blue light and blends them together in varying intensities to create different colors. With that said, it is important to note that a digital camera carries the same subjective values as the human eye and might not always be an accurate means to assess a patient's tooth shade (see chapter 4).

Reflective and transmissive media: CMY(K) color model

Media such as printed materials and photographs are considered *reflective*, and media such as slides and transparencies are considered *transmissive*, because, respectively, they are visualized through the reflection of light off of their surfaces and the transmission of light through their surfaces as previously described. Color

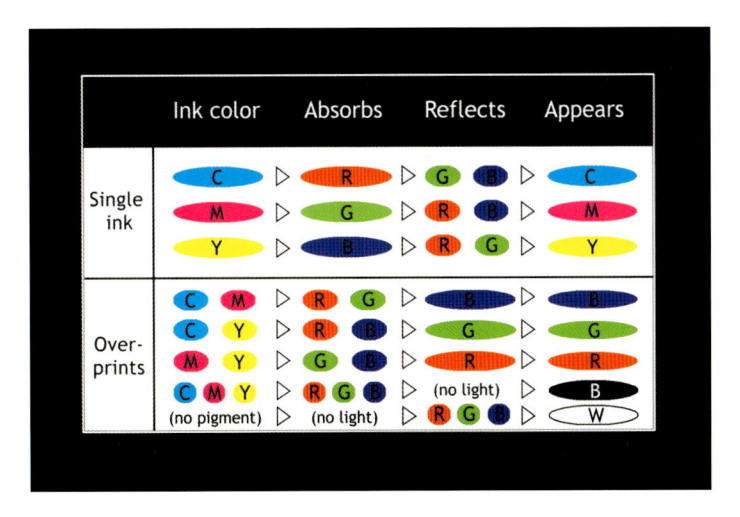

Fig 1-17

Subtractive primary colors. Subtractive primaries are formed when one additive primary is absorbed and the remaining two are reflected. For example, cyan is formed when the additive primary color red is absorbed and the remaining two additive primary colors, green and blue, are reflected.

reproduction in reflective and transmissive media is based on the color-absorbing qualities of materials such as ink or dyes. These materials are formulated to absorb some wavelengths and reflect/transmit others to create specific colors. The primary colors in these color systems are those created by the absorption of one of the RGB wavelengths and the reflection/transmission of the others. They are referred to as *cyan*, *magenta*, and *yellow* (CMY). Cyan is produced when red is absorbed and green and blue are reflected/transmitted; *magenta* is produced when green is absorbed and red and blue are reflected/transmitted; and *yellow* is produced when blue is absorbed and red and green are reflected/transmitted. The absence (or *subtraction*) of these three colors would mean that no wavelengths could be absorbed and therefore all wavelengths would be reflected/transmitted, resulting in the color white. For this reason, cyan, magenta, and yellow are referred to as the *subtractive primary colors*: Color is created by *subtracting* (absorbing) certain numbers of RGB wavelengths (Fig 1-17).

Conversely, the presence of all three colors (CMY) should result in all wavelengths being absorbed and none reflected/transmitted, ie, the color black. Although this is true for CMY dyes used in photography, use of all three colors

1 Color Theory

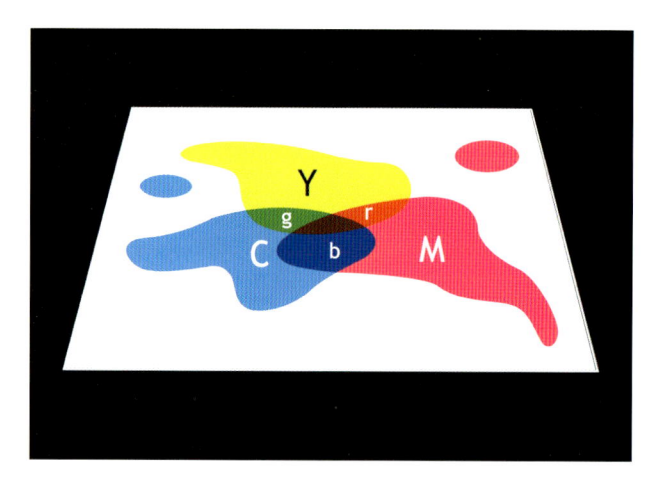

Fig 1-18
Subtractive primaries are used in color printing.

of printing ink will actually result in a muddy brown because of inherent imperfections in the ink. Therefore, black (indicated by *K* in order to differentiate it from blue [*B*]) ink is usually added to improve the appearance of darker colors and to create better shadow density, which is why *CMYK* and *four-color processing* are the terms usually associated with full-color printing[11] (Fig 1-18).

Color in Dentistry

Once the processes of color perception and reproduction are well understood, they can be applied to dentistry, specifically to shade-matching techniques. The important concepts include pigment colors (similar to the subtractive colors discussed above) and the dimensions of color that must be considered when matching shades.

Pigment colors

Pigment colors are the inherent hues of an object. Because these colors are perceived through either transmission or reflection of light, they are essentially the same as the subtractive colors used in color reproduction for reflective and transmissive media, as discussed above. In dentistry it is imperative to understand pigment colors since they are inherent in restorative materials (eg, ceramics, com-

Color in Dentistry

Table 1-3 Pigment Colors

Primary color	Secondary/complementary colors
Red	Green
Yellow	Violet
Blue	Orange

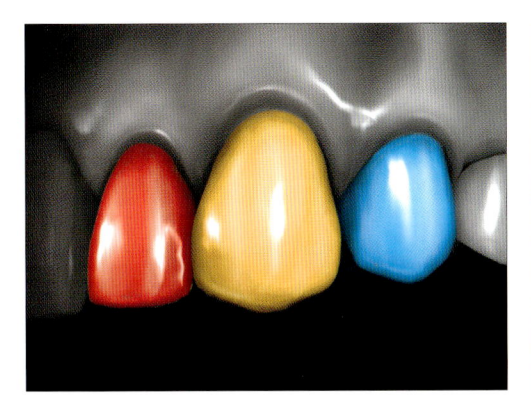

Fig 1-19
Pigment colors are directly related to the subtractive primary colors, but are referred to as *red*, *yellow*, and *blue*.

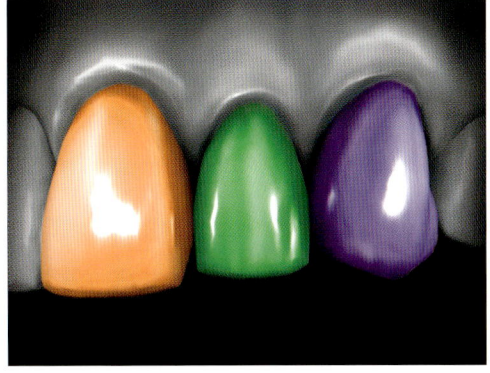

Fig 1-20
Secondary pigment colors (orange, green, and violet) are formed when two primary pigment colors are added together.

posites, and acrylic resins). Moreover, understanding primary, secondary, and complementary colors is critical to achieving accurate, esthetic shades (Table 1-3).

Primary colors: Red, yellow, blue

The primary pigment colors are very similar to the subtractive primaries, but they are referred to as *red*, *yellow*, and *blue*, rather than *magenta*, *yellow*, and *cyan*, respectively (Fig 1-19). Like the subtractive primaries, these are the colors that are perceived when one of the RGB wavelengths is absorbed: red is perceived when green is absorbed; yellow is perceived when blue is absorbed; and blue is perceived when red is absorbed.

Secondary colors: Orange, green, violet

The secondary colors are formed by combining two of the primary colors: red and yellow create orange; yellow and blue create green; and blue and red create violet (Fig 1-20).

13

1 Color Theory

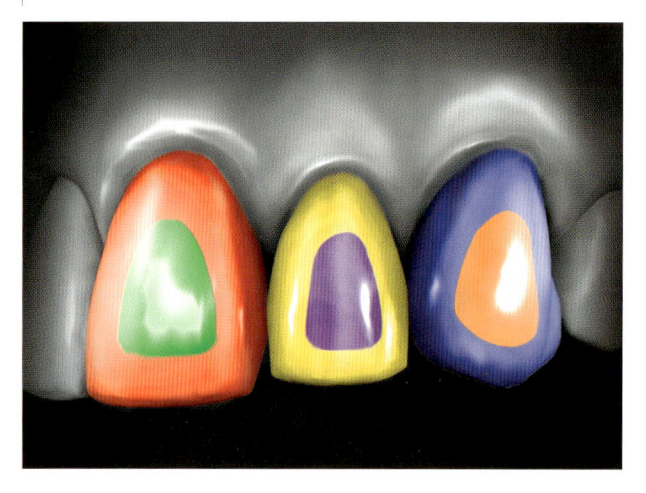

Fig 1-21
Complementary colors: red/green, yellow/violet, and blue/orange.

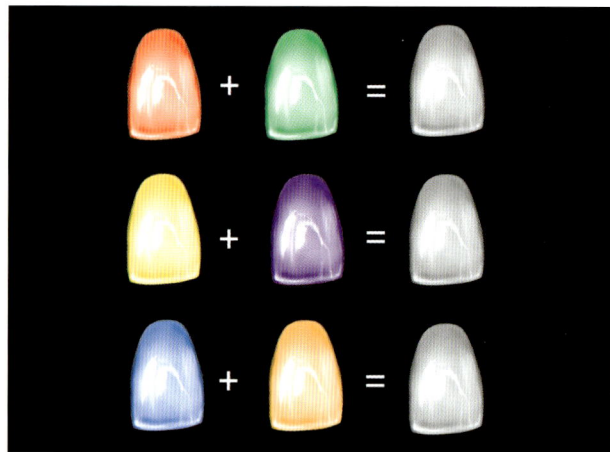

Fig 1-22
When complementary colors are added together, they neutralize each other and form gray. This is clinically significant because complementary colors can be combined to lower the value of excessively bright restorations.

Complementary colors

Complementary colors are so named because they "go well" together; these are the colors often seen paired in advertising (Fig 1-21). Complementary colors are those that, when combined in equal proportions, will form a dull gray that absorbs and reflects/transmits all wavelengths in equal amounts (Fig 1-22). The complementary pigment color pairs are blue/orange, red/green, and yellow/violet.

The additive principle of complementary colors may be used to alter the value of restorations. For example, if the value of a restoration needs to be lowered, the complementary color can be added to that restoration to make the shade more gray and hence lower in value (eg, shade A3 contains an orange hue; therefore, adding blue stain will create a lower value).

Dimensions of color

Like the teeth and restorations we are trying to match, color is truly multidimensional. At the beginning of the 20th century, Professor Albert H. Munsell noted that each color has a logical relationship to all other colors.[12] He brought clarity to color communication by establishing an orderly system for accurately identifying every color. This "color wheel" includes the dimensions of *hue*, *value*,

Color in Dentistry

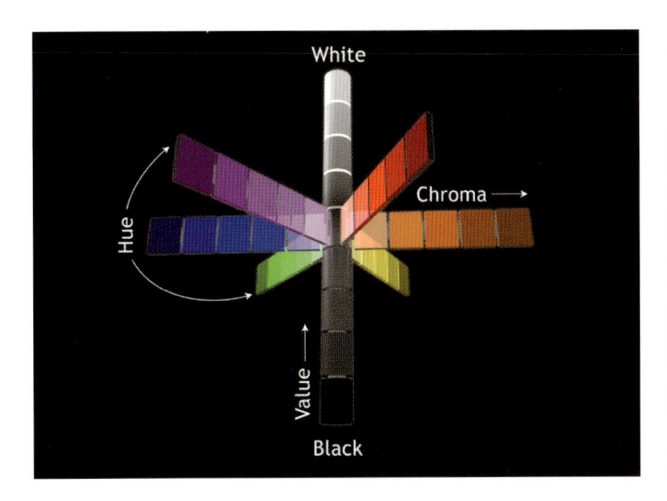

Fig 1-23
Munsell's color wheel. Color is described in terms of hue, chroma, and value.

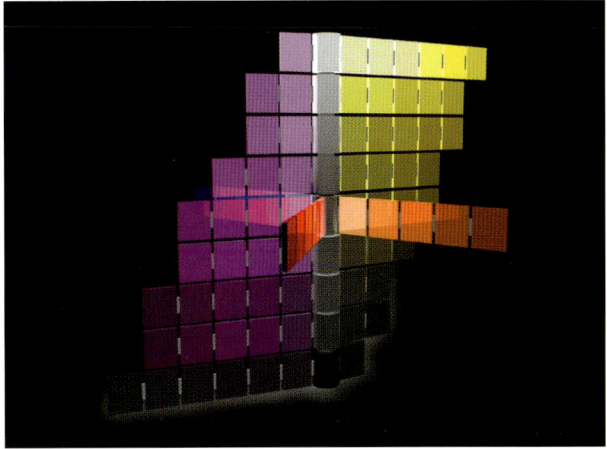

Fig 1-24
Munsell's color wheel in three dimensions. The shape of the wheel is skewed toward the red-purple colors since humans are visually more sensitive to these colors.

TABLE 1-4 COLOR DIMENSION TERMINOLOGY

Term	Dimension of color
Hue	Color tone
Chroma	Saturation/purity of color
Value	Relative lightness/darkness of color

and *chroma* (Figs 1-23 and 1-24; Table 1-4). To these dimensions should be added *translucency*, which is not addressed in Munsell's color analysis but is perhaps the most critical factor in the quest for an esthetic restoration. The four dimensions are defined as follows:

- Hue: Synonymous with the term *color*. Used to describe the pigments of a tooth or dental restoration (eg, red, blue, or yellow).
- Value: The relative darkness or lightness of the hue. The greater the total amount of light reflected, the higher the value. The scale of value ranges from a low of 0 for pure black to high of 10 for pure white.
- Chroma: The intensity or saturation and purity of the color tone (hue). The more wavelengths of a particular color that are reflected (relative to all other

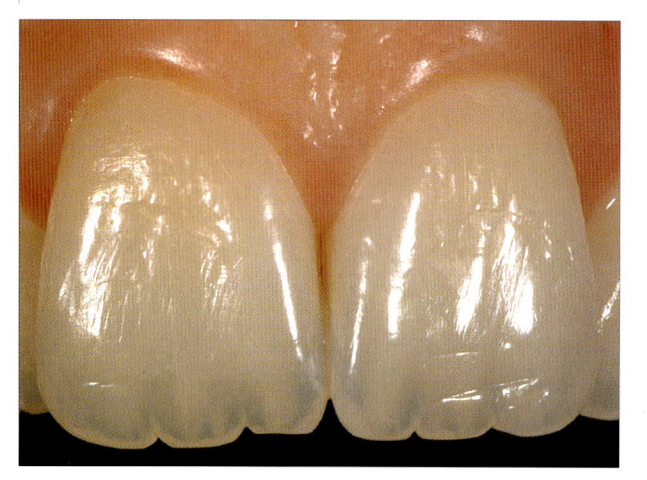

1 Color Theory

Fig 1-25
Maxillary central incisors with bluish incisal translucency.

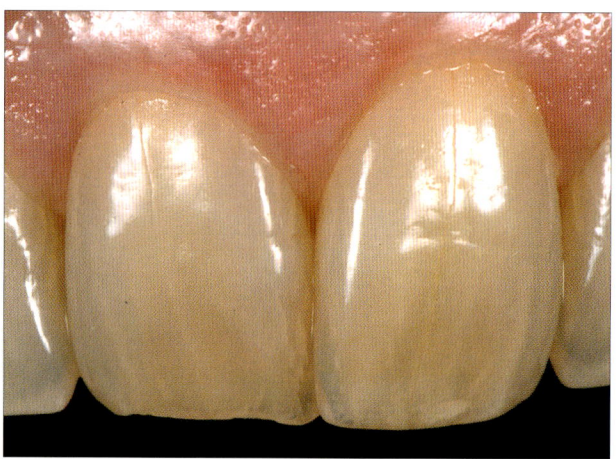

Fig 1-26
Maxillary central incisors with bluish-orange incisal translucency due to aging.

color wavelengths), the higher the chroma of that hue (ie, the color is deeper and more pure).

- Translucency: The degree to which light is transmitted rather than absorbed or reflected. The highest translucency is transparency (ie, all light is transmitted), while the lowest is opacity (ie, all light is reflected or absorbed). The incisal edges of natural teeth are translucent, and accurate translucency determination is vital to a restoration's esthetic success (Figs 1-25 and 1-26). A mistake in translucency will greatly compromise the natural appearance of a restoration. Although there is currently no method for quantifying translucency in the clinical setting, lab technicians can use a densitometer to measure the amount of light that is transmitted through a restoration or shade tab.

Trained laboratory technicians generally can determine value and hue when presented separately. However, difficulties arise when value and chroma are coupled together, resulting in inconsistencies in value determinations for dental restorations.[13]

It is recommended that clinicians use an 18% gray card (available at most photographic supply retail outlets) as a background when viewing shade tabs and teeth to eliminate distractions in the surrounding environment and allow a more accurate determination of chroma and value (see chapter 5).

Summary

- Each individual perceives color differently.
- A full range of colors can be very closely simulated using the dominant colors: red, green, and blue.
- Control and understanding of the composition of colors is critical when attempting to alter a shade.
- Munsell defined the dimensions of color as hue, value, and chroma. However, in dentistry, translucency is of equal importance.

References

1. A Guide to Understanding Color Communication. Grandville, MI: X-Rite, 2002.
2. Hunter RS, Harold RW. The Measurement of Appearance. New York: Wiley, 1987:3–68.
3. Judd DB, Wyszecki G. Color in Business, Science and Industry, ed 3. New York: Wiley, 1975.
4. Kuehni RG, Marcus RT. An experiment in visual scaling of small color differences. Color Res Appl 1979;4:83–91.
5. Chu SJ. The science of color and shade selection in aesthetic dentistry. Dent Today 2002;21(9):86–89.
6. Berns RF. Billmeyer and Saltzman's Principles of Color Technology, ed 3. New York: Wiley, 2000:75–104.
7. Commission Internationale de l'Eclairage. Colorimetry, Official Recommendations of the International Commission on Illumination [Publication CIE No. 15 (E-1.3.1)]. Paris: Bureau Central de la CIE, 1971.
8. Miller L. Organizing color in dentistry. J Am Dent Assoc 1987;115(special issue):26E–40E.
9. Wyszecki G, Stiles WS. Color Science Concepts and Methods, Quantitative Data and Formulae, ed 2. New York: Wiley, 1982:83–116.
10. Bunting F. The ColorShop Color Primer. Available at: http://www.xrite.com/documents/mktg/ColorPrimer.pdf. Accessed 18 September 2003.
11. Miller MD, Zaucha R. Color and tones. In: The Color Mac: Design Production Techniques. Carmel, IN: Hayden, 1992:23–39.
12. Munsell AH. A Grammar of Color. New York: Van Nostrand Dreinhold, 1969.
13. Chu SJ. Precision shade technology: Contemporary strategies in shade selection. Pract Proced Aesthet Dent 2002;14:79–83.

2 Elements Affecting Color

In this chapter:
- Illumination and clinical lighting conditions
- Contrast effects and optical illusions
- Impact of viewer's physical and mental state on color perception
- Importance of restorative material selection

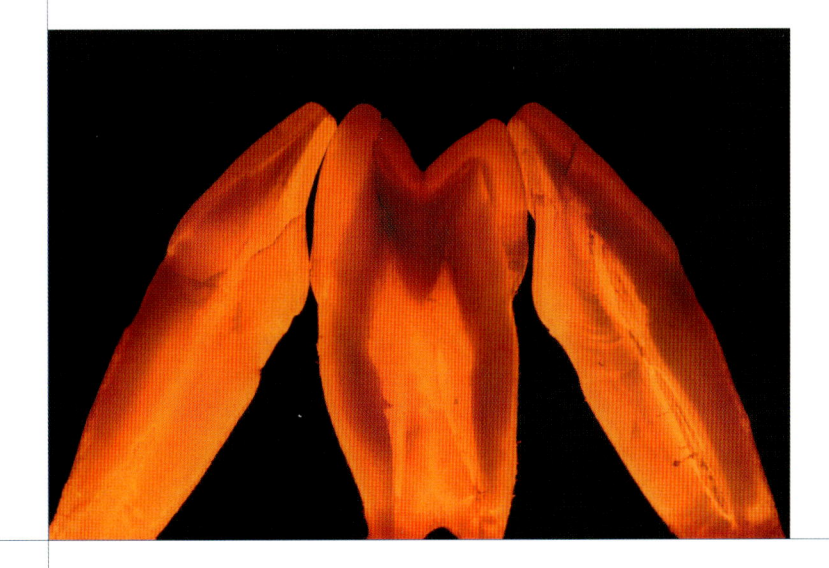

2 Elements Affecting Color

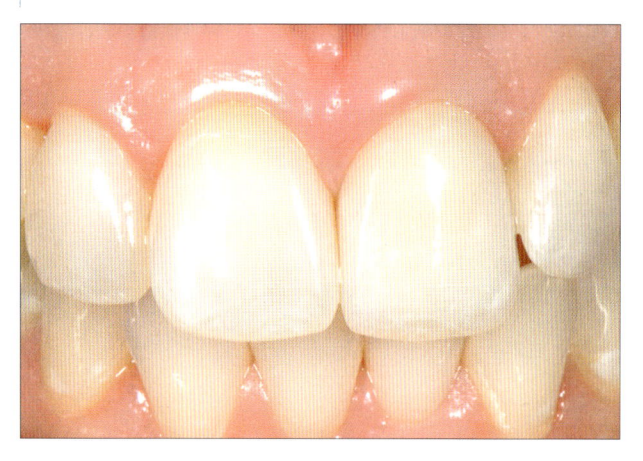

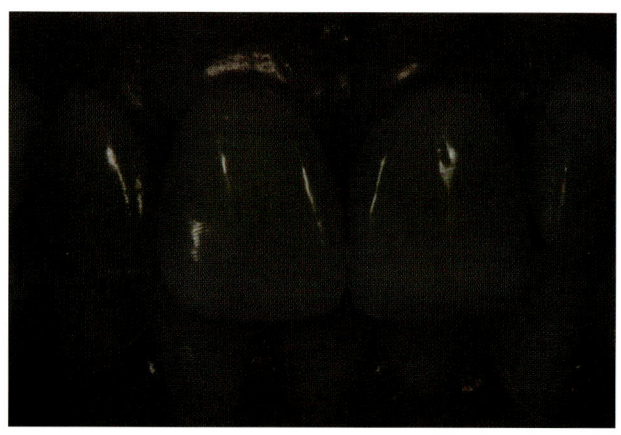

Fig 2-1
Too much illumination obliterates detail necessary for accurate shade matching.

Fig 2-2
Insufficient illumination makes it difficult to discern tooth shades.

There are many variables that affect how a color is perceived. For example, the color of the ocean cannot carry a blanket description of *blue*. The ocean appears to be a different color at night than it does at midday, with varying hues at different levels of relative lightness and brightness. The surrounding scenery, such as the sky, beach, and vegetation, can create contrasts that affect the perceived color of the waters. Moreover, different viewers may perceive the ocean as being different colors even when viewing it under the same conditions. The same rules apply in the dental operatory during shade-matching procedures. The lighting conditions, the environment, and the viewer all play vital roles in color perception and evaluation.[1]

Illumination

Color can be neither accurately perceived nor correctly evaluated without proper illumination. It is not only crucial to have enough lighting to evaluate color properly (Figs 2-1 and 2-2), but it is also essential to achieve the proper quality of lighting. This is accomplished by using the correct light intensity and the proper illuminants. However, even when these variables are well controlled, there are certain clinical challenges associated with lighting and shade matching that must be considered.

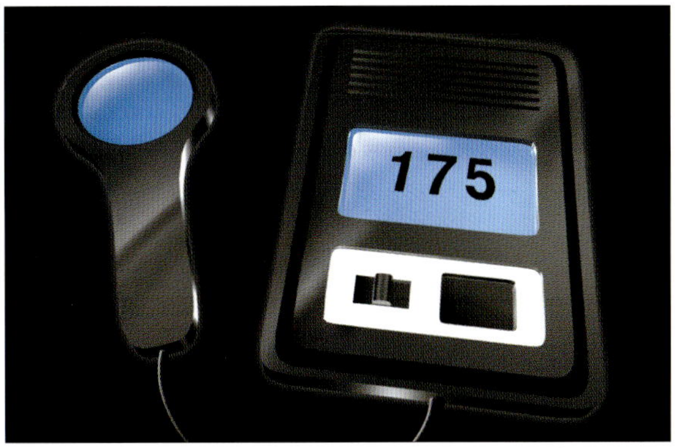

Fig 2-3
A light meter can be used to assess the proper quantity of light (150 to 200 foot-candles) in the dental operatory.

Light intensity

The intensity of light is the most common regulator of pupil diameter, which is a crucial factor in accurate shade matching.[2] The accurate identification of color is only determined at the center of the visual field, ie, what is perceived by the fovea. The fovea is located in the center of the retina and contains a high concentration of cone cells, which provide the greatest visual acuity and most accurate color perception. Much of the rest that is perceived is "synthesized" by the visual cortex of the brain.[3] Therefore, the most accurate color reading is obtained by the human eye when the pupil is opened enough to fully expose the cones in the fovea. This is achieved by maintaining a lighting intensity of 150 to 200 foot-candles, as verified by a light meter (Fig 2-3).

Maintaining a lighting intensity of 150 to 200 foot-candles (as verified by a light meter) will facilitate accurate shade analysis and matching.

Standard illuminants

The type of illuminant used can significantly impact the perception of color. A system created in 1931 by the *Commission Internationale de l'Éclairage* (CIE; translates to International Commission on Illumination) categorized illuminants based on their effect on color perception.[4] This system was developed to allow manufacturers of products such as paints and inks to specify and com-

2 Elements Affecting Color

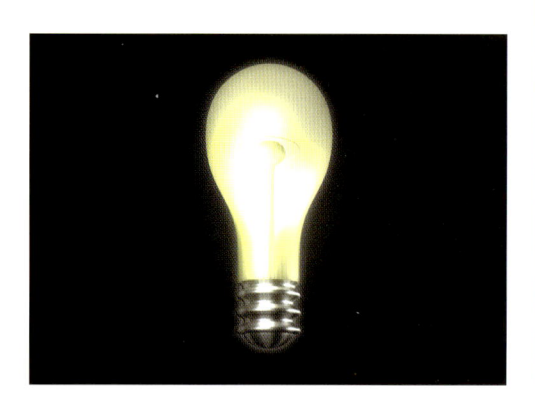

Fig 2-4
Illuminant A represents incandescent lighting conditions with a color temperature of about 2,856 K.

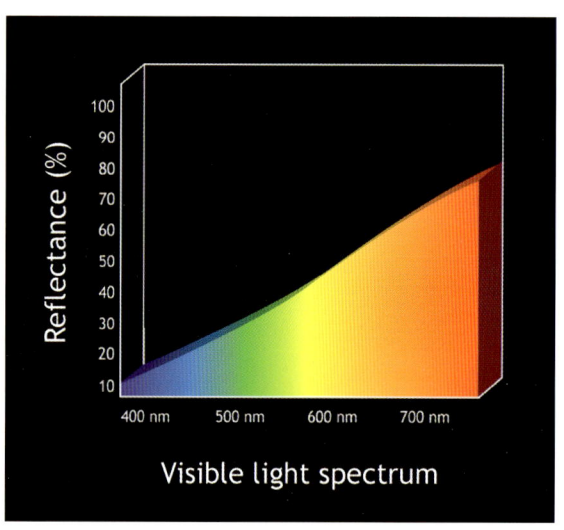

Fig 2-5
Spectral reflectance curve for illuminant A.

municate the colors of their products. In their report, the CIE designated three standard illuminants, A, B, and C, to which they later added a series of D illuminants, a hypothetical E illuminant, and, unofficially, a series of fluorescents (F). Following is a brief summary of the A through F illuminants[5]:

- A: A tungsten light source with a correlated temperature of about 2,856 K, producing a yellowish-red light (Figs 2-4 and 2-5). Generally used to simulate incandescent viewing conditions (eg, household light bulbs).
- B: A tungsten light source coupled with a liquid filter to simulate direct sunlight with a correlated temperature of about 4,874 K (Fig 2-6). Rarely used today.
- C: A tungsten light source coupled with a liquid filter to simulate indirect sunlight with a correlated temperature of about 6,774 K (Fig 2-7). Used in many viewing booths because indirect sunlight is considered a common viewing condition. However, illuminant C is not a perfect simulation of sunlight because it does not contain much ultraviolet light (required when evaluating fluorescence).
- D: A series of illuminants representing different daylight conditions, as measured by color temperature. Illuminants D_{50} and D_{65} (so called because their

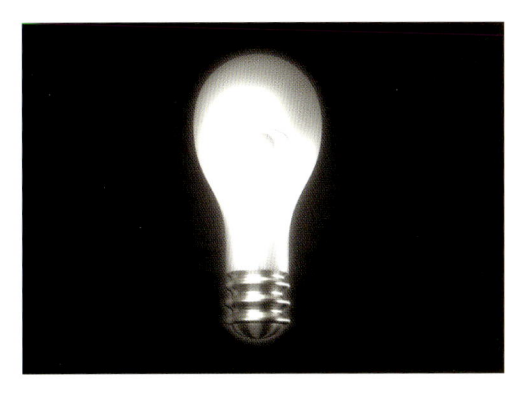

Fig 2-6
Illuminant B represents direct sunlight at about 4,874 K.

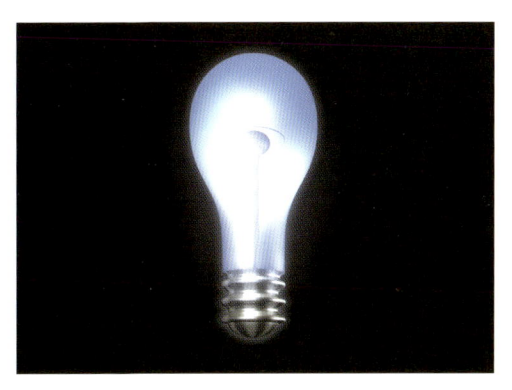

Fig 2-7
Illuminant C represents indirect sunlight at about 6,774 K.

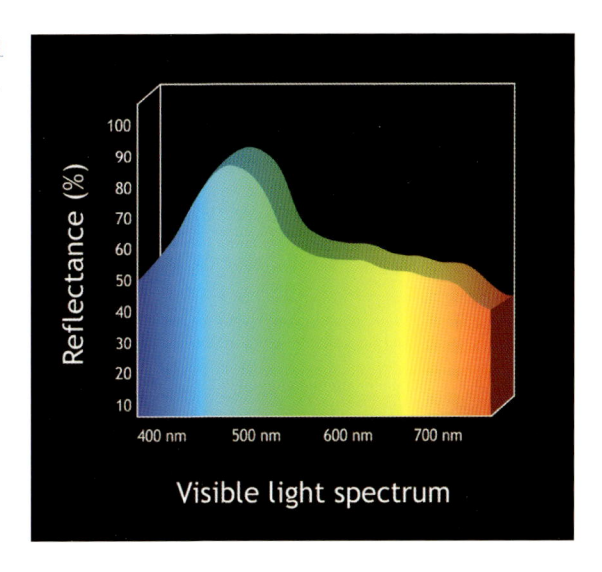

Fig 2-8
Spectral reflectance curve for D_{50} illuminant, representing bluish daylight conditions.

correlated color temperatures are 5,000 and 6,500 K, respectively) are commonly used as the standard illuminants for graphic arts viewing booths and correspond to bluish daylight reflectance (Fig 2-8). Illuminant D_{65} is nearly identical to illuminant C except that it is a better simulation of indirect sunlight because it includes an ultraviolet component for better evaluation of fluorescent colors.

2 Elements Affecting Color

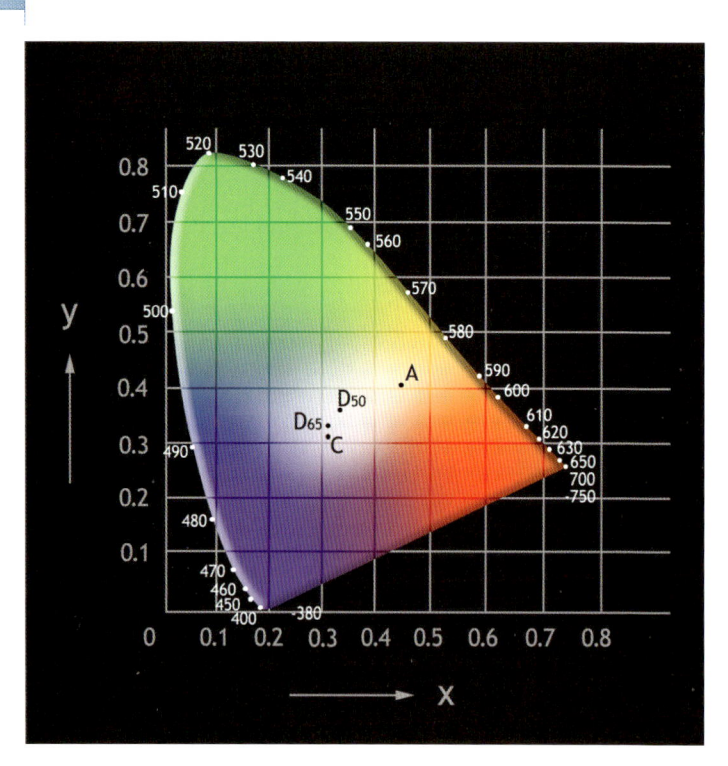

Fig 2-9
Chromaticity diagram with plotted points representing illuminants A, C, D_{50}, and D_{65}. The diagram shows the distribution of color that the cones of the human eye can perceive (human eye sensitivity), based on the CIE color coordinates *x* and *y*. The cones are more sensitive to purples and reds versus yellows and greens, as demonstrated by the teardrop shape of the diagram's color distribution.

- E: A theoretical light source with equal amounts of energy at each wavelength. This illuminant does not actually exist, but is a useful tool for color theorists.
- F: A series of fluorescent light sources. Because fluorescent lights have sharp peaks in their spectral curves and thus defy definition by color temperature, they are not officially considered standard illuminants. However, since viewing conditions using fluorescent lighting are common, the CIE recommends certain light sources for evaluating colors destined for fluorescent environments.

These illuminants are represented in color calculations as spectral data (Fig 2-9). The spectral reflectance power of light sources, which are emissive objects, is really no different from the spectral data of a reflective colored object. The hue, chroma, and value of different types of light sources can be recognized by examining their relative power distribution as spectral curves (Figs 2-10 to 2-13).

When performing shade matching, clinicians should use D_{50} illuminants, which provide the closest lighting rendition to natural sunlight in respect to illumination *quality* and *quantity* and therefore present the best opportunity to see and select the correct shade.

ILLUMINATION

Fig 2-10
The location of the rise of a light source's spectral reflectance curve relative to wavelength indicates its hue. Note the rise in the red wavelength for vibrant red light and the spike in the curve in the green wavelength for dark green light.

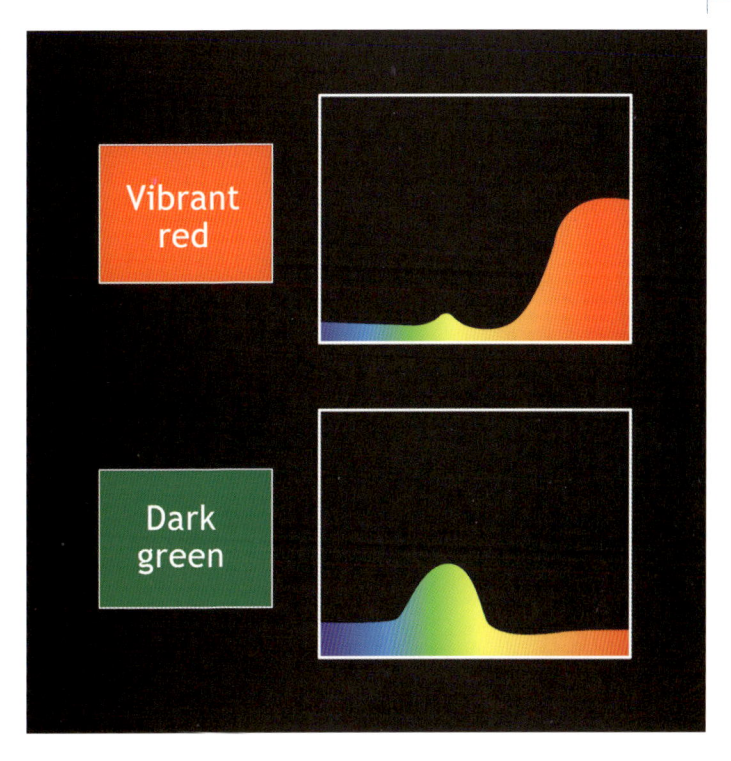

Fig 2-11
The purity of the curve or the distinctiveness of the shape of the curve determines the saturation, or chroma, of the light. The more uniform the shape of the curve, the lower the light's chroma.

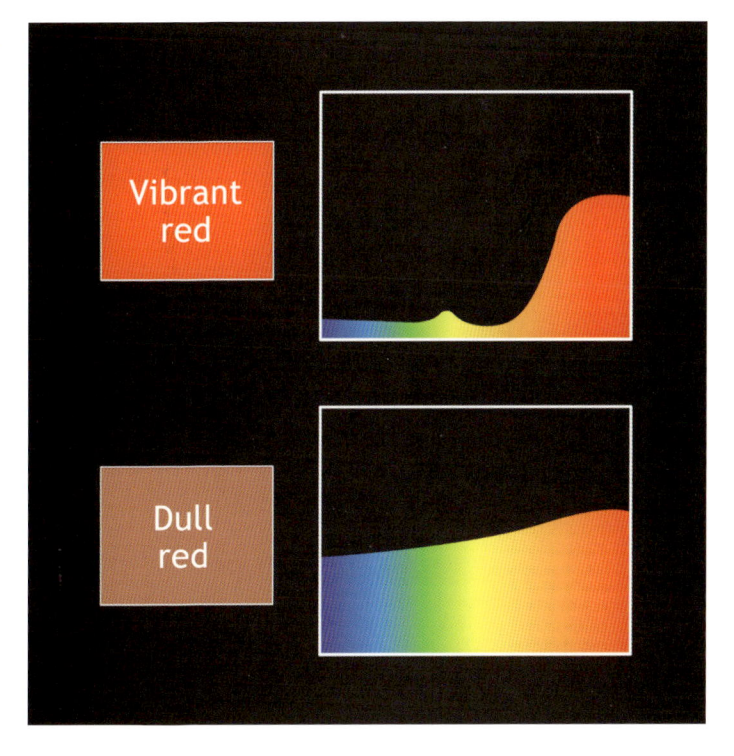

25

2 Elements Affecting Color

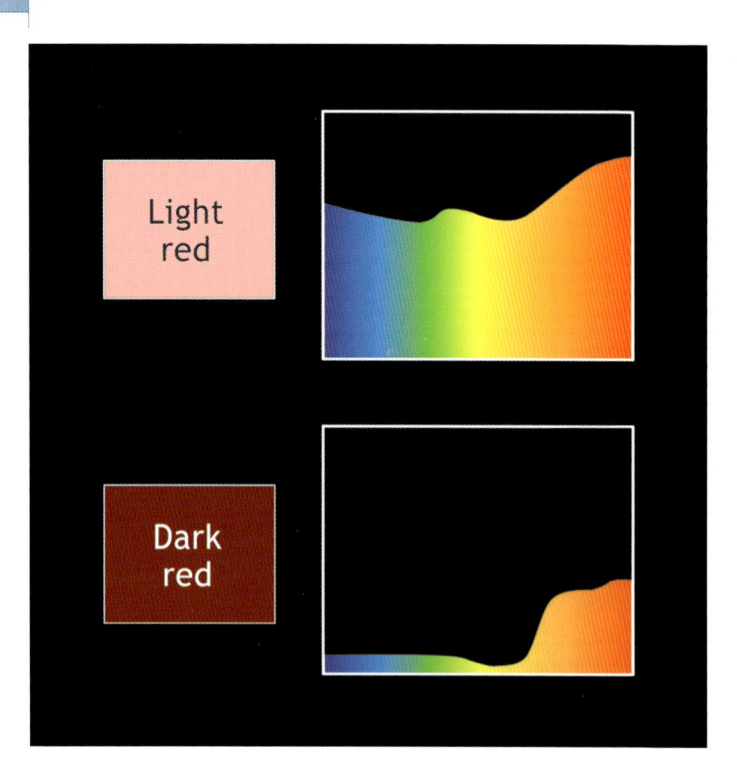

Fig 2-12

The amplitude, or height, of the curve's waves determines the value of the light. The higher the curve, the higher the value (ie, the brighter the light).

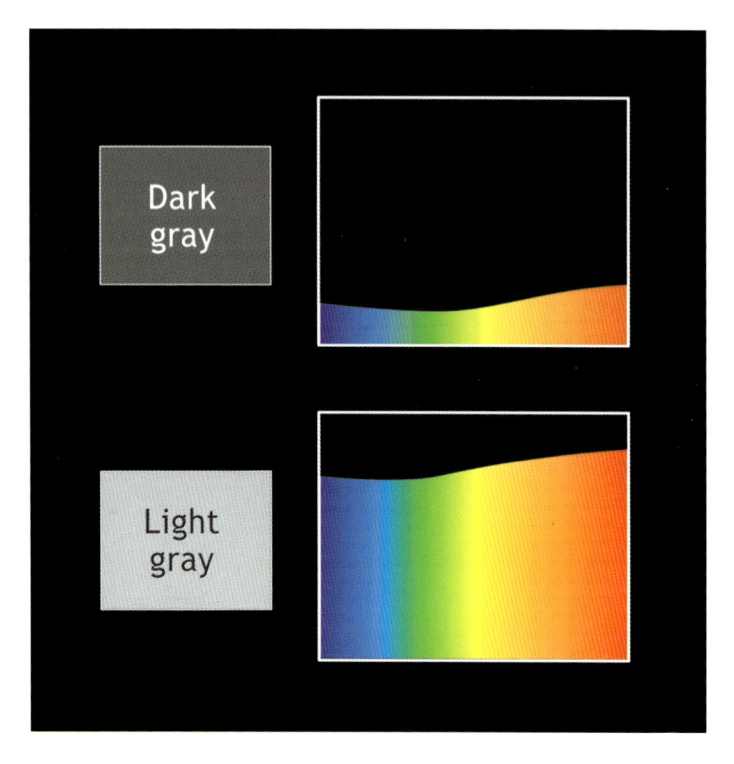

Fig 2-13

The uniformity of these spectral curves indicates the low chroma and absence of a distinct hue that characterize gray-colored light. The difference in amplitude indicates whether the gray light is low in value (dark) or high in value (light).

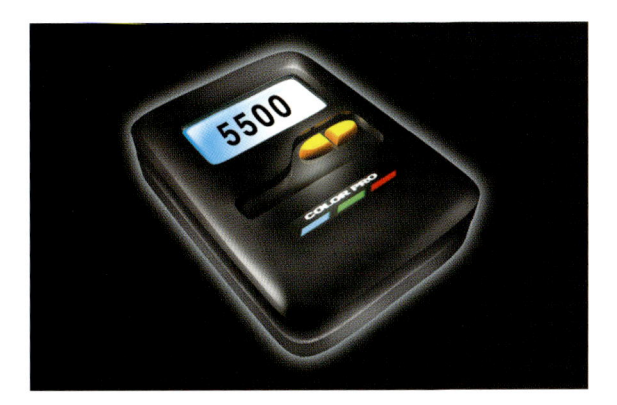

Fig 2-14
A color temperature meter, which measures lighting quality. The proper color temperature for the dental operatory is about 5,500 K.

Clinical lighting challenges

Dental professionals have long relied on so-called color-corrected lighting when evaluating tooth shade, yet using lights with that particular designation does not ensure accurate color matching.[2] As discussed below, the reason for this is twofold: *(1)* conflicts in lighting and *(2)* metamerism.

Lighting conflicts

The dental operatory is not free from conflicts in lighting. Light coming in through a window mixes with the fluorescent light coming from the hallway and the color-corrected lighting in the dental operatory. Amid these various lighting conflicts, it is the job of the clinician to analyze the opposing teeth and to determine an accurate shade match. The following tips[6] will aid in that process.

- If the clinician or the lab technician has access to a natural light source, it is best to perform shade matching at 10 AM or 2 PM on a clear, bright day when the ideal color temperature of 5,500 K is present.
- Color-corrected lighting tubes that burn at about 5,500 K (D_{50} illuminants) should be installed when only artificial lighting is available (ie, when there is no natural light).
- A color temperature meter should be used periodically to verify that a color temperature of 5,500 K is achieved in the shade-matching area (treatment room or surgery) (Fig 2-14).
- Dust and dirt should be cleaned routinely from lighting tubes and diffusers because the presence of dust may alter the quantity and quality of emitted light.

2 Elements Affecting Color

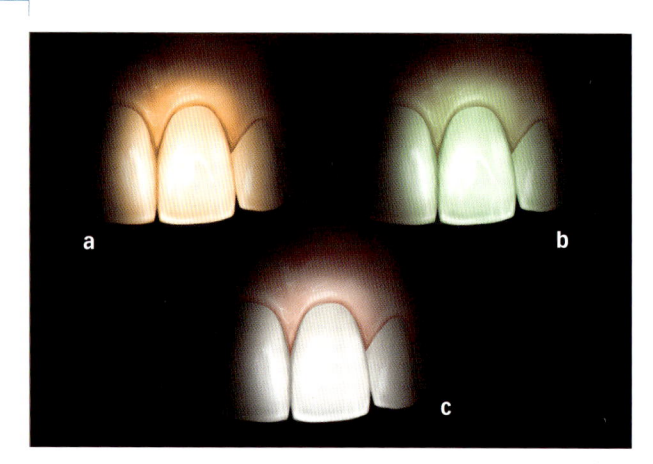

Fig 2-15
Illustration of the effect on perceived color if the proper lighting quality is not used. (a) Incandescent lighting (2,856 K). (b) Fluorescent lighting (4,000 K). (c) Color-corrected lighting (5,500 K).

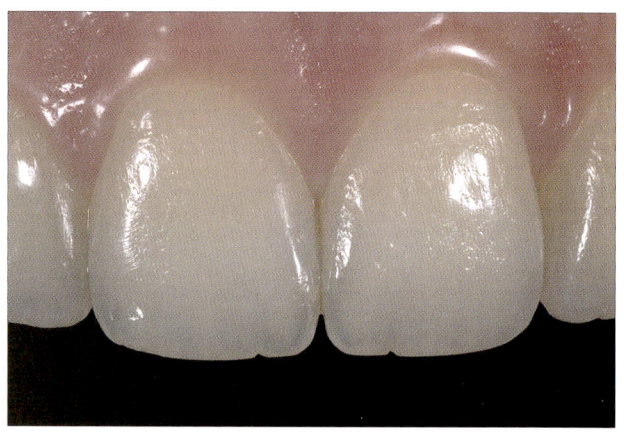

Fig 2-16
A ceramic tooth viewed under sunny daylight conditions (approximately 5,200 to 5,500 K; D_{50} illuminant).

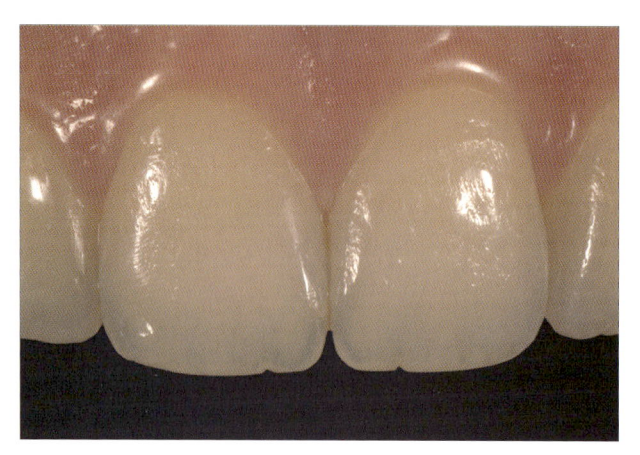

Fig 2-17
The ceramic tooth shown in Fig 2-16 viewed under tungsten lighting (approximately 2,856 K; illuminant A).

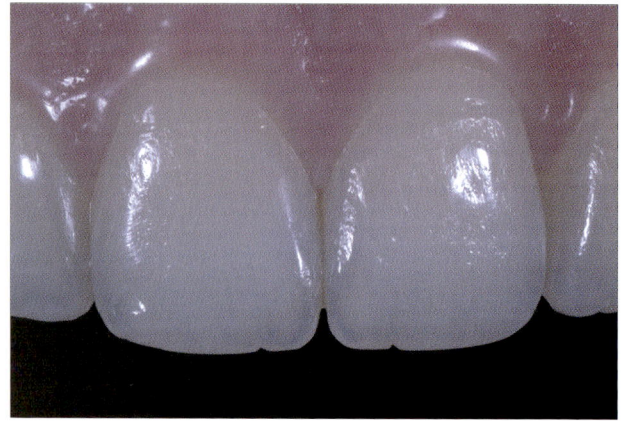

Fig 2-18
The ceramic tooth shown in Figs 2-16 and 2-17 viewed under fluorescent light (approximately 4,000 K; illuminant F).

Metamerism

Color-corrected lighting is designed to match the wavelengths and relative quantity of visible light coming from the sun; however, a person's smile will be viewed under any number of different lighting conditions, causing restorations to appear completely different in terms of hue, value, and chroma (Figs 2-15 to 2-18). Like the restorations themselves, traditional shade tabs will appear different when viewed under various lighting conditions, creating difficulties in shade matching.

ILLUMINATION

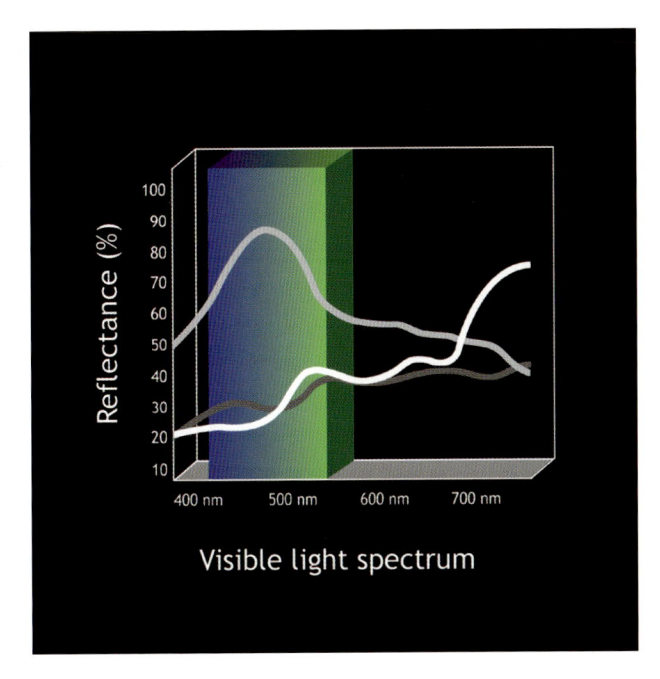

Fig 2-19
Spectral curves for light source approximating daylight conditions *(gray line)* and two gray objects *(white and black lines)*. Note that the objects appear to match under these lighting conditions (the two spectral curves intersect at around 500 nm).

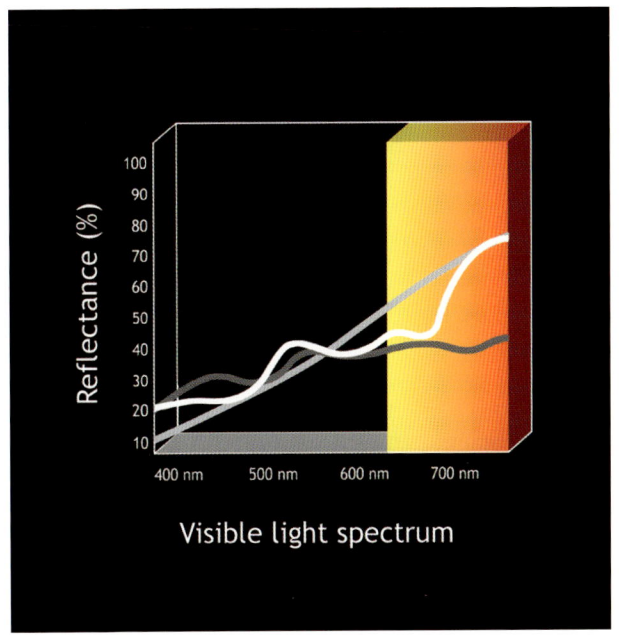

Fig 2-20
Spectral curves for warm, reddish incandescent light source *(gray line)* and the same two gray objects *(white and black lines)*. Note that under these lighting conditions the two objects are no longer a visual match (ie, metamerism occurs) as the spectral curves diverge significantly at 700 nm.

The phenomenon of two objects appearing to match in color under one condition but showing apparent differences under another is termed *metamerism*. This is known in some circles as the "jacket and pants problem." What can appear to be perfectly matched under the fluorescent lighting of a clothing store can look significantly different in natural light. The two objects are referred to as a *metameric pair*. In dental terms, metamerism occurs when a crown is matched to the natural dentition under incandescent light, but, when viewed under color-corrected or fluorescent light, appears not to match the natural teeth. This can occur frequently, and mistakes can often be glaring, resulting in a return visit, an unhappy patient, and unproductive chair time. However, the only sure way to avoid metamerism is to achieve a spectral curve match. Pairs of colored objects that have the same spectral curve will always match regardless of the light in which they are viewed. Advanced technology in dentistry has greatly increased the chances of achieving a spectral curve match (see chapter 4). Pairs of colored objects that do not have the same spectral components may or may not match under different lighting conditions (Figs 2-19 and 2-20).

2 Elements Affecting Color

Fig 2-21 Clinical appearance of a crown on the maxillary left central incisor under color-corrected lighting conditions (quantity: 175 foot-candles; quality: 5,500 K).

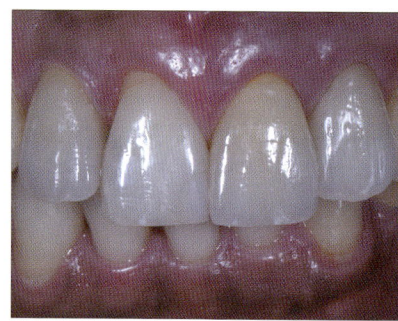

Fig 2-22 Same crown shown in Fig 2-21 under fluorescent lighting. Note that the crown appears to match better under this type of light versus color-corrected lighting.

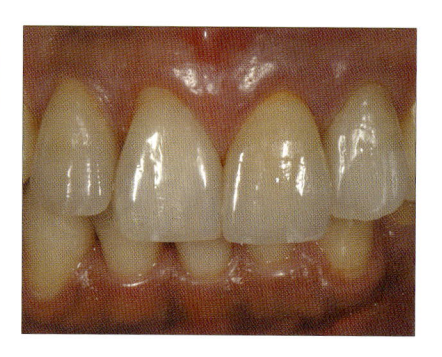

Fig 2-23 Same crown shown in Figs 2-21 and 2-22 under incandescent light. The crown least appears to match the surrounding dentition under this lighting.

Although some manufacturers have tried to combat metamerism by developing materials that exhibit a chameleon effect by taking on the color of their surroundings, metamerism continues to be a problem in the dental operatory (Figs 2-21 to 2-23). Metamerism complicates shade selection and, on the whole, can only be recognized and explained. With all variables being equal, there is often no solution to it. Therefore, clinicians must explain to patients that in some situations a restoration may not match as well as in others and that this is an *occurrence*, not a *fault*.[7]

To combat metamerism, the clinician can perform shade selection and assessment (verification) under various lighting conditions. However, because some degree of metamerism is generally unavoidable, the clinician should explain to the patient that it is natural for the color of restorations to vary slightly under different lighting conditions.

Contrast Effects

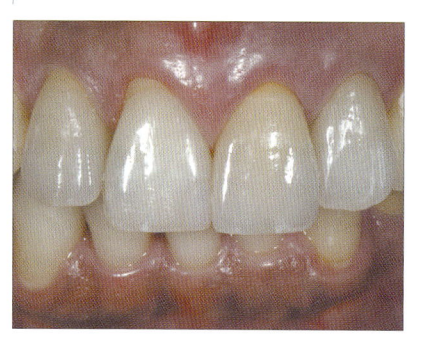

Contrast effects are visual phenomena that can alter considerably the perception of color, as well as the ability to evaluate color in a clear, concise, and objective way. These effects create optical illusions that are difficult to decipher unless the observer is prepared for them. The different categories of contrast effects are described in the following text and summarized in Table 2-1.

TABLE 2-1 CLINICAL SIGNIFICANCE OF CONTRAST EFFECTS

Contrast effect	Clinical effect	Clinical application
Value	Correlated to surrounding environment, ie, skin tone, hair color, eye color, and the value of the adjacent dentition and periodontium. A darker environment will make a tooth appear lighter and vice versa.	Select lighter shades for patients with lighter tones and darker shades for those with deeper tones in the dentofacial area. Err toward the value tendency of the surrounding dentition (ie, low value if dentition is dark, high value if dentition is light).
Hue	The complementary color of the surrounding background or environment is more apparent in the tooth.	Use a light blue or neutral gray (18%) background card when selecting shades to eliminate surrounding distractions and to precondition the eyes for improved perception of complementary color tones.
Chroma	A less chromatic background will make the tooth color appear more intense and vice versa. Also, a background with a hue and chroma similar to that of the tooth will make it difficult to discern the tooth shade.	Use background cards with a lower chroma (eg, gray) relative to the shade of the tooth to make the tooth shades more intense and therefore easier to discern.
Areal	Large teeth appear lighter; light teeth appear larger; small teeth appear darker; dark teeth appear smaller.	If a restoration appears too large, consider decreasing the value by half a shade.
Spatial	Recessed teeth appear darker; dark teeth appear more recessed; protrusive teeth appear lighter; light teeth appear more protrusive.	Recessed teeth can be made lighter; protruding teeth can be made darker. Consider orthodontic therapeutic correction, bleaching, or conservative esthetic restoration.
Successive	When one color is viewed immediately following another, an afterimage often will appear and affect perception of the second color.	Take breaks between looking at different shades to avoid the effects of afterimages.

Simultaneous contrast

Simultaneous contrast occurs when two colors are observed at the same time. When perceiving more than one color at once, the brain will attempt to achieve a harmonic balance of the colors. Perception of the color therefore is affected by three factors: *(1)* the surrounding relative lightness (the color will appear to be darker in lighter surroundings and vice versa); *(2)* the surrounding color (the color will appear to have shifted toward its surrounding color's complement); and *(3)* the surrounding relative saturation (the color will appear to be more intense

2 Elements Affecting Color

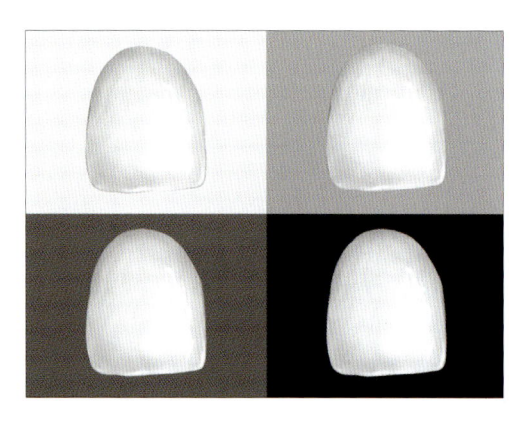

Fig 2-24
Value contrast effect. The same tooth appears increasingly lighter as the backgrounds become darker.

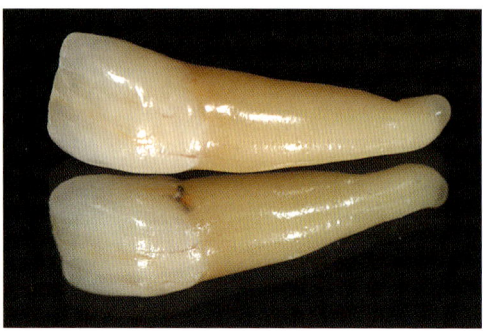

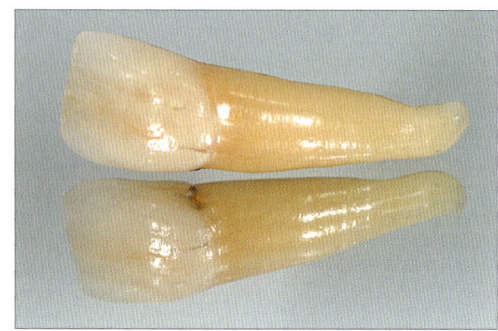

Figs 2-25 and 2-26
A ceramic tooth appears lighter against a dark background (Fig 2-25) than it does against a lighter background (Fig 2-26).

in less chromatic surroundings and vice versa). Identical colors will appear to be different when framed by different backgrounds or patterns in reference to lightness, color, and saturation. These effects are referred to as *value contrast*, *hue contrast*, and *chroma contrast*, respectively.[8]

Value contrast

Visual judgment of lightness is not dependable, primarily because the relative lightness of an object is affected by the lightness of the contrasting background or surroundings. For example, if the surrounding background is dark, an object will appear light. However, if the same object is placed against a lighter background, it is perceived as darker (Figs 2-24 to 2-26). What this illustrates is that the perceived lightness can vary, even though the reflectivity of the object is constant. This is due to the fact that the retina is very sensitive to light. It expands and contracts in response to varying light intensities as they are interpreted by the brain. If the background is darker than the object, the retina must adapt to

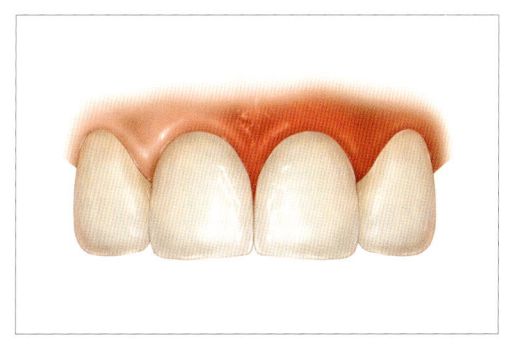

Contrast Effects

Fig 2-27
Value contrast effects have clinical significance when dealing with excessively inflamed gingival tissues. The dark value of the inflamed gums will trick the eyes into perceiving the tooth shade as being lighter than it actually is. As a result, the fabricated restoration will appear too dark once the tissues have healed.

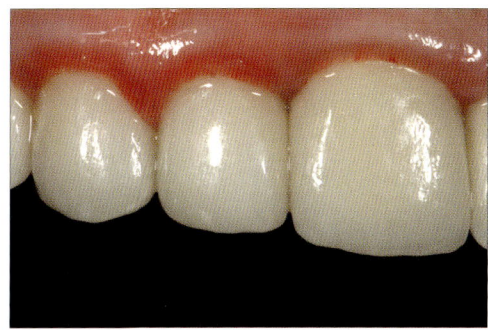

Fig 2-28
A common clinical scenario of excessively inflamed gingival tissues due to either periodontal disease or violation of the biologic width. To avoid errors caused by value contrast effects, shade-matching procedures should not be performed until such inflammation has been resolved.

the relatively lighter object, causing the brain to perceive it as lighter than if the object were viewed by itself. If the background is lighter than the object, the opposite effect results. However, because the eye adapts much more quickly from dark to light than from light to dark, the effect of a darker object on a lighter background will always be more pronounced.

A practical dental example of this phenomenon is when a restoration is viewed adjacent to inflamed gingival tissues (Figs 2-27 and 2-28). The redness (darkness) of the gingivae (background) distorts color perception, making the restoration (object) appear lighter than it actually is. As a result, a crown that is too low in value (ie, dark) may be chosen. The mistake becomes apparent when the tissues heal and the crown appears darker than the adjacent teeth.

To combat value contrast effects in dental restorations, relatively lighter shades should be selected for patients with light-toned surrounding dentition and soft tissues, while darker shades should be chosen for patients with darker pigmentation in the dentition and soft tissues, since teeth will appear darker in contrast with lighter tones and lighter in contrast with darker tones.

Hue contrast

A color will be perceived differently when viewed in conjunction with various background or adjacent colors with contrasting hues. For example, a tooth or

2 Elements Affecting Color

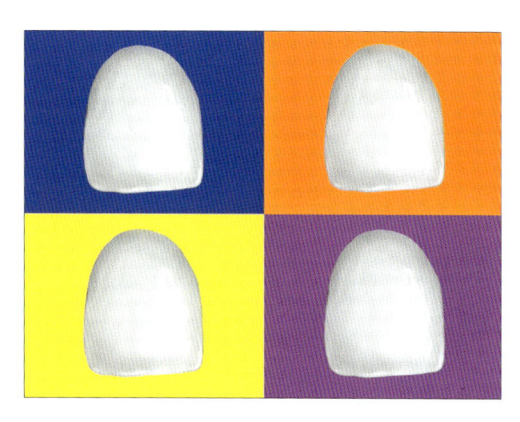

Fig 2-29
Hue contrast effect. When viewed against different background colors, the teeth appear to take on the hue of the background's complementary color.

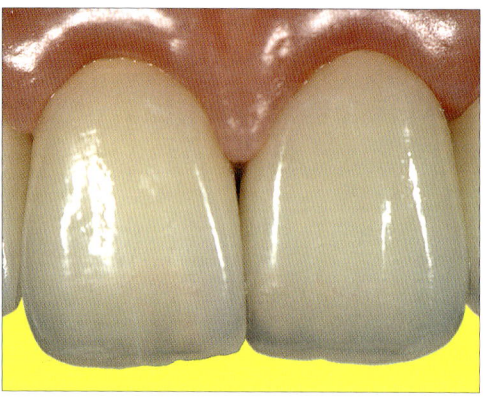

Fig 2-30
The yellow background causes the ceramic veneer restorations to take on a purple cast when viewed for a prolonged period of time.

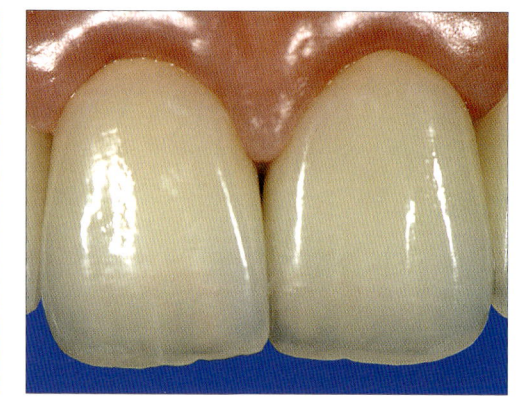

Fig 2-31
The same ceramic veneers shown in Fig 2-30 appear orange in hue because of the blue background.

restoration will appear bluish against an orange background and purplish if the background is yellow (Figs 2-29 to 2-31). When a color is viewed simultaneously with another color, the perceived hue of the first color will appear more similar to the complementary color of the second color. Using this contrast effect, dental professionals can precondition their eyes when taking shades by first looking at a complementary color, then looking at the tooth shades. This will allow the clinician to see the color of the tooth shades more effectively.

A majority of tooth shades fall into the orange hue family.[7] To view the orange tones with a more critical eye, dental professionals can precondition their eyes by looking at a light blue shade immediately prior to the shade selection process. The closer the tooth shades are to the complementary color (ie, light orange), the more vibrant they will appear.

Contrast Effects

Fig 2-32
Chroma contrast effect. The highly chromatic tooth appears more vibrant against the background that is low in chroma and less vibrant against the background that closely matches the chroma of the tooth.

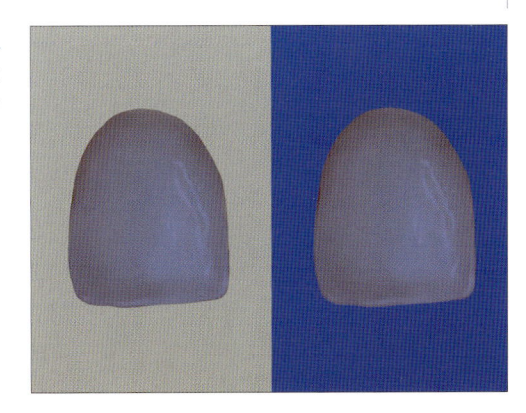

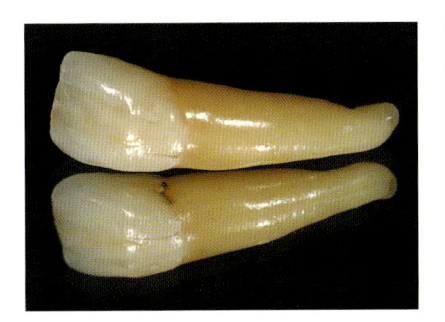

Fig 2-33
A ceramic tooth without influence of background chroma effects.

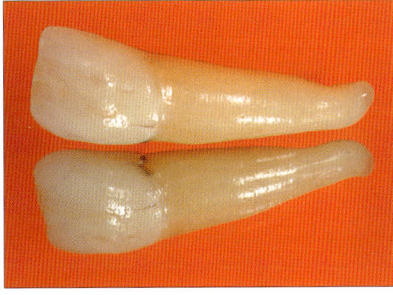

Fig 2-34
Ceramic tooth shown in Fig 2-33 against an orange background. Note that the tooth is less visible against a background similar in chroma.

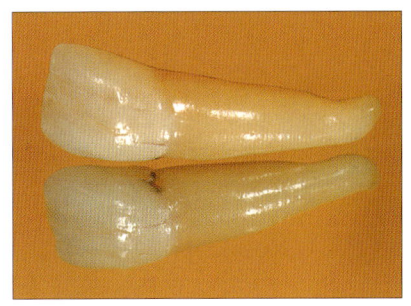

Fig 2-35
Ceramic tooth shown in Figs 2-33 and 2-34 against a yellow background. The tooth is even less visible against a background that very closely approximates its chroma.

Chroma contrast

This contrast follows the same effect as the value and the hue contrasts. An object will appear more intense against a background low in chroma, and less intense against a more chromatic background (Fig 2-32). In addition, the closer the object is to the hue and chroma of the surrounding background, the less visible it becomes. This is important to remember during shade matching; using backgrounds of similar hue and chroma to the teeth will make it more difficult to distinguish the shade (Figs 2-33 to 2-35).

2 Elements Affecting Color

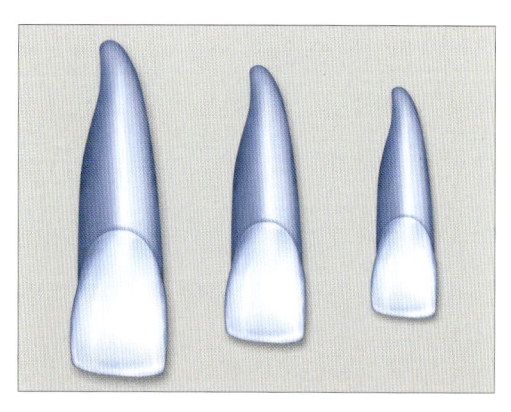

Fig 2-36
Areal contrast effect. A larger image appears lighter since the surface area is greater and reflects more light back to the observer. Conversely, a smaller object is less reflective and appears darker.

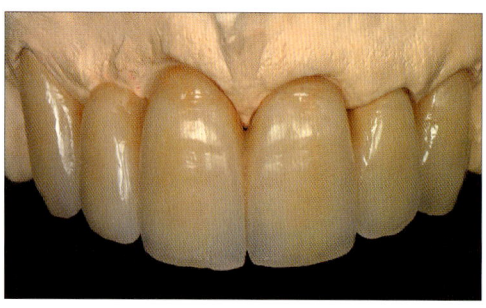

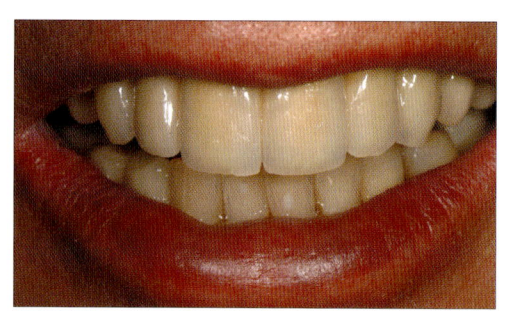

Figs 2-37 and 2-38
Clinical case of very large maxillary central incisors as part of a fixed partial prosthesis. Even though all of the teeth are the same shade (Vita A3), the central incisors appear lighter because of areal contrast effects.

Areal contrast

The size of the object can also influence visual color perception. For instance, a larger object will appear lighter than a smaller object of the same color. Likewise, a lighter object will appear to be larger than a darker object of the same size (Fig 2-36). This type of contrast accounts for the fact that darker clothes have a tendency to make an individual look smaller and thinner, while lighter clothes tend to make the individual appear larger and heavier.

If teeth or restorations appear too large, consider decreasing the value (Figs 2-37 and 2-38). If they appear too small, the value may be increased by one half the shade. Teeth or restorations that appear darker than the surrounding dentition because of a smaller size may be lightened with a bleaching or whitening procedure or by replacing the restoration.

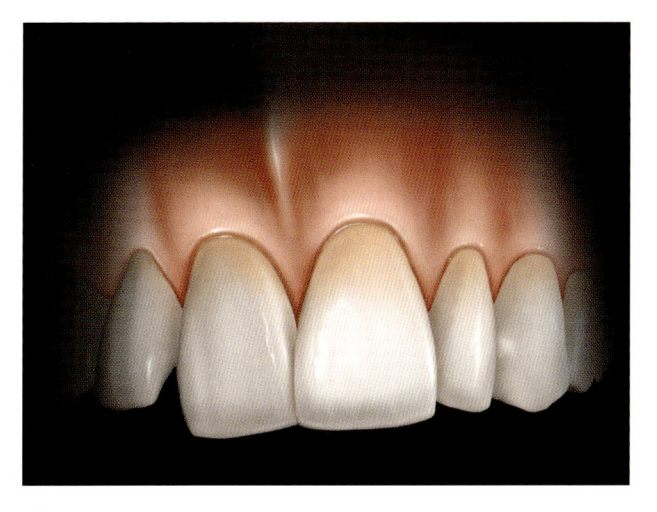

CONTRAST EFFECTS

Fig 2-39
Spatial contrast effect. Teeth that are rotated and/or recessed relative to the adjacent teeth appear to be darker.

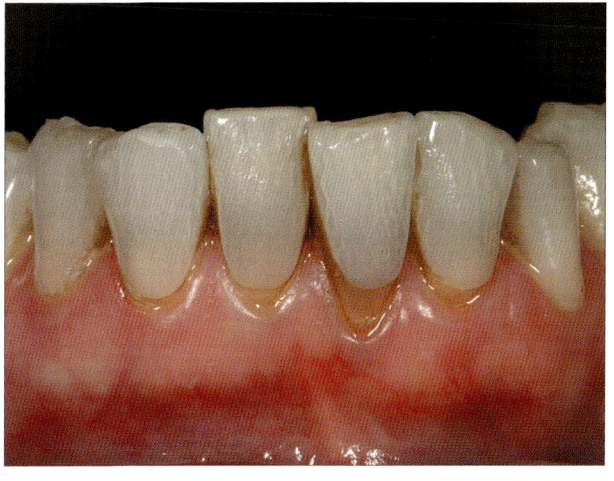

Fig 2-40
Clinical example of spatial contrast. The mandibular right central incisor appears darker than the other teeth because of its recessed position.

Spatial contrast

An object closer to the observer will appear larger and lighter, whereas an object more recessed will appear to be smaller in size and darker (Fig 2-39). This phenomenon is frequently seen with rotated and overlapped teeth. The recessed teeth appear to be darker (Fig 2-40). Posterior teeth also appear to be darker, and the shadows in the mouth further contribute to this appearance.

When determining the shade of a restoration, the clinician should maintain the same distance from the patient's mouth in order to get a consistent reading. To compensate for spatial contrast, recessed teeth can be made lighter, and protruding teeth can be made darker.

Successive contrast

Successive contrast occurs when one color is viewed following the observation of another color. The visual perception remains after the eye has left the object. Afterimages are categorized as positive (similar) or negative (different). Positive afterimages have the same color as the original perception; negative afterimages have the opposite, or complementary, color to the original perception.

2 Elements Affecting Color

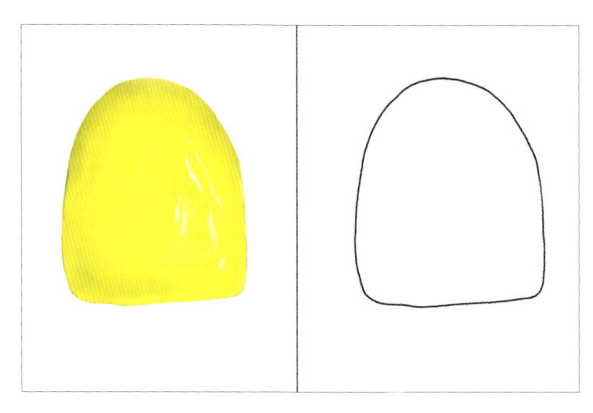

Fig 2-41
Successive contrast effect. A positive (similar) or negative (complementary) afterimage of the colored tooth will be seen in the blank tooth after brief or long visual contact, respectively, with the colored tooth.

Positive afterimages occur following a short visual interaction, while negative afterimages occur after long visual contact with an object (Fig 2-41). The latter is caused by depletion of the neurotransmitter rodopsin in the cones of the retina during prolonged staring, which makes it physically impossible to see that particular color.

Understanding how color perception can potentially deviate because of various contrast effects allows the clinician to select a shade more effectively. With a solid understanding of how opposing and adjacent colors can play tricks on the interpreter, the chances for an accurate shade match can be dramatically improved.

Viewer-Associated Effects

Color blindness

A person with color blindness has trouble seeing red, green, blue, or mixtures of these colors. The term *color vision problem* is often used instead of *color blindness* because most people with color blindness can see some color. Although the condition might be perceived as rare, approximately 10% of US

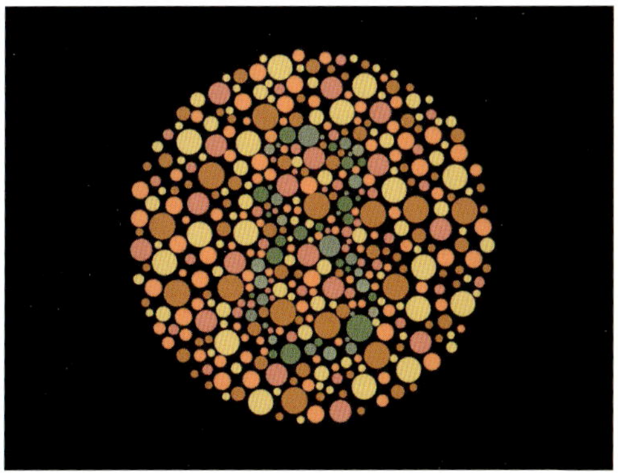

Fig 2-42
Color blindness test to assess levels of sensitivity to green and yellow. The number 8 should be visible.

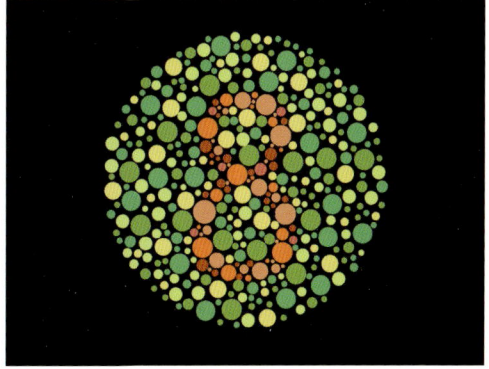

Fig 2-43
Reversed color blindness test. The number 8 is more easily seen because its purple-red color is easily detected by the cones of the eyes.

males (but only 0.3% of US females) are affected by color blindness.[9] Most optical exams include tests for color blindness (Figs 2-42 and 2-43).

Color blindness is caused by a deficiency in or absence of one or more of the three types of photosensitive pigments able to detect red, green, and blue. These pigments are contained in the photosensitive cells in the human eye that allow color perception. These cells are called *cones* and are located in the center of the retina. The essential effect of color blindness is that hues that appear different to most people look the same to those with color blindness. In other words, having a color vision deficit means that the ability to discriminate hue, saturation, and lightness is reduced (although lightness is less affected since the rods are responsible for that part of visual color discrimination). This is a serious problem for a clinician performing shade matching since determining the hue, value, and chroma of a restoration is critical to its natural appearance.

Age

Aging is detrimental to color-matching abilities because the cornea and lens of the eye become yellowed with age, imparting a yellow-brown bias and causing the differentiation between white and yellow to become increasingly difficult. This process begins at age 30, becomes more noticeable after age 50, and has clinical significance after 60 years of age. After age 60, many people have significant difficulties in perceiving blues and purples.[10,11]

2 Elements Affecting Color

Fatigue

Tired eyes cannot perceive colors as accurately as alert eyes can. Compromised visual perception is the consequence of systemic, local, and/or mental fatigue. The inability to accurately determine hue and chroma is most evident during times of fatigue; in addition, color may be perceived as faded or blurry. Successive shade observations (ie, treating many patients requiring shade assessment during a single workday) can be one of the primary causes of fatigue. Fatigue is the most common cause of an inaccurate shade match.

When evaluating multiple consecutive shades, the dental professional should take a brief break between restorations. This will help avoid the problems associated with both successive contrast and fatigued eyes and thereby ensure greater success in achieving an accurate shade match.

Nutrition

An individual's eating habits play an important role in the health of the eye. Some scientists have suggested that there is an association between macular degeneration (a physical disturbance of the center of the retina [called the *macula*] causing gradual loss of vision) and a large intake of substances high in saturated fat.[12] There is also evidence that eating fresh fruits and dark green, leafy vegetables may delay or reduce the severity of macular degeneration. Additionally, supplementation with antioxidants such as vitamins C and E has been shown to have positive effects in slowing the progression of the disease in some cases. Other trace minerals and nutrients such as zinc and lutein are also important for the health of the eyes.[13] An individual's nutrition is an essential factor in the overall health of the body, and the eye is certainly no exception.

Emotions

Color can function as a language. For example, in many places throughout the world, red suggests anger or passion, yellow represents joy, and blue is associated with sadness. Without delving into the complexity of the human emotional tie to color, it is worthwhile to note the following scientific evidence, which is of significance to the dental professional.

It is generally known that emotion can affect pupillary diameter, causing dilation or constriction, and, as stated in the previous discussions about light

TABLE 2-2 EFFECT OF CHEMICALS ON COLOR PERCEPTION		
Drug	Effect on red/orange/yellow	Effect on blue/green/purple
Alcohol or morphine	Lighter	Darker
Caffeine	Darker	Lighter

intensity and value contrast, pupillary diameter has a direct effect on color discrimination. Additionally, it has been shown that in the practice of meditation a subject can be trained to control brain wave patterns to favor certain waves; when in meditation, people report the appearance of colored halos around objects, as well as other alterations of visual perception. It is therefore clear that regardless of how a color may affect a person's mood, the initial mood or mental state of the observer can be a critical factor in color determination.[14]

Medications

The abuse of drugs, alcohol, and caffeine will affect not only judgment, but also color perception (Table 2-2). In addition, many prescription and even over-the-counter medications are associated with visual side effects. Medications can act on any part of the visual system from the visual cortex to the retina. Like all drug side effects, they vary from person to person. Some side effects are neither predictable nor apparent to the individual taking the medication. It is safe to assume that most clinicians will take some medication in their lives, and the older people get the more likely they are to take multiple medications. Viagra, a drug used to treat erectile dysfunction, is notorious for causing vision to have a blue tint, which makes it difficult to distinguish between blue and green. As a result of these findings, the Federal Aviation Administration now requires all commercial airline pilots to refrain from the consumption of Viagra 12 hours prior to flight time.[2]

Of special concern for female practitioners are the side effects caused by oral contraceptives, ie, red-green or yellow-blue discrimination defects. They also can cause a blue tinge, and there are several studies that indicate that long-term use of oral contraceptives will cause a decrease in color perception of blues and yellows.[15]

2 Elements Affecting Color

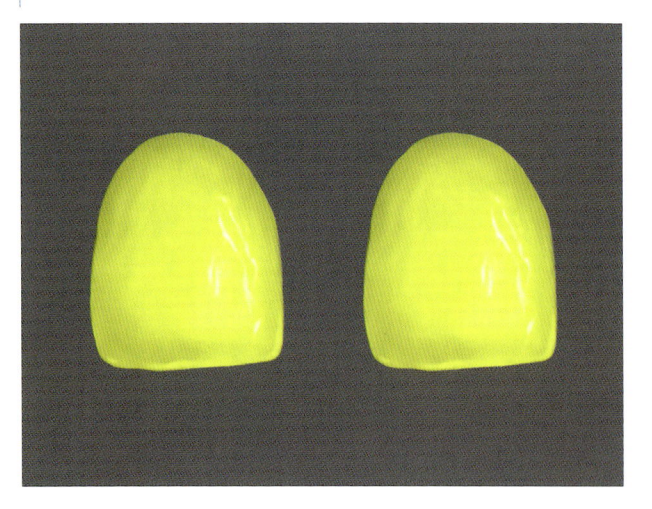

Fig 2-44
Binocular difference in color perception. When two objects of the same shape and color are arranged side, by side they may appear to be different, eg, one may seem to be slightly lighter than the other.

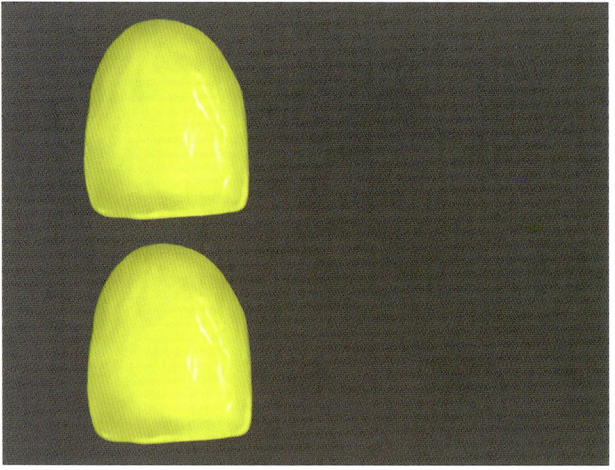

Fig 2-45
If the two objects are placed on the same side, the effect is not evident.

Binocular difference

Binocular difference is the perception difference between the right eye and the left eye. It often becomes evident during an eye exam when a person can see the vision chart better with one eye than the other. It is also not uncommon for color blindness tests to be conducted during a routine eye examination to establish the patient's deficiencies in each eye. While color disparity between a person's eyes is relatively minor, one should be aware of it and, if necessary, compensate for it. To check for binocular color difference, two objects are placed side by side under uniform illumination. They may appear different, eg, the one on the right may seem slightly lighter than the one on the left. A binocular color difference exists if the object on the right still appears lighter when the placement is altered (Figs 2-44 and 2-45).

Placing shade tabs either above or below (rather than next to) the tooth to be matched will help to eliminate error caused by binocular difference.

Restorative Materials Selection

Fig 2-46
Clinical photograph taken in natural light of two extracted teeth *(center and right)* and one all-ceramic tooth replica *(left)*. Materials that allow technicians to mimic the natural appearance of human teeth are presently available.

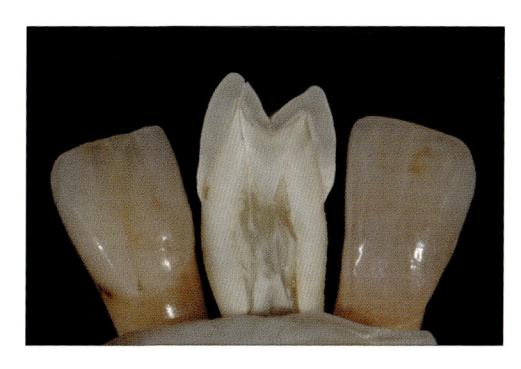

Fig 2-47
The same teeth shown in Fig 2-46 under reflected light. The properties of the ceramic tooth are similar to those of the natural teeth.

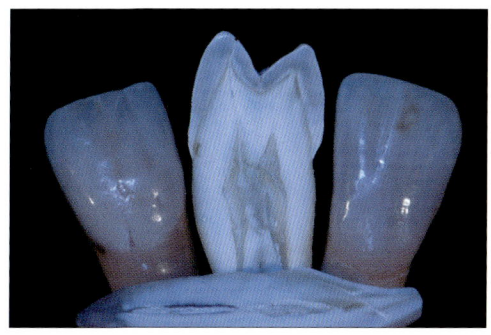

Fig 2-48
The same teeth shown in Figs 2-46 and 2-47 under transmitted light. The ceramic tooth exhibits the same translucency as the natural teeth.

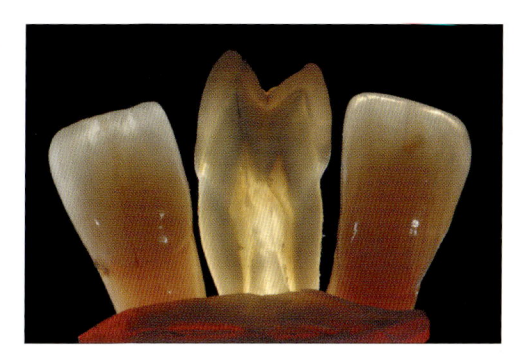

Restorative Materials Selection

The choice of restorative material is extremely important for achieving an accurate shade. The relative translucency of the tooth to be matched and the material selected must coincide (Figs 2-46 to 2-48). Bleached teeth can be especially problematic to match (Fig 2-49). This is because their color is achromatic: Hue is white; chroma is low (ie, there is little saturation of hue); and value is high (ie,

2 Elements Affecting Color

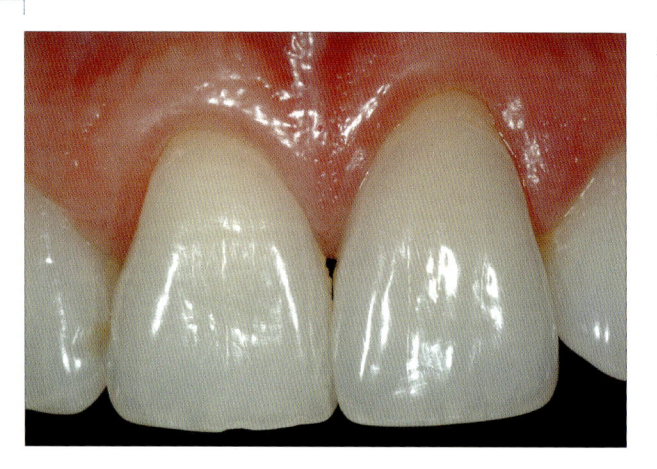

Fig 2-49
Bleached teeth can be challenging to match because they are achromatic, ie, devoid of hue and chroma, leaving value as the only visual parameter.

TABLE 2-3 FRACTURE TOUGHNESS AND RELATIVE OPTICAL PROPERTIES OF MATERIALS FOR CERAMIC LAMINATE VENEER RESTORATIONS

Material	Brand names	Flexural strength (MPa)	Translucency
Slip-cast alumina ceramics	In-Ceram (Vita, Bad Sackingen, Germany)	630	Low
High-alumina-reinforced (sintered) ceramics	Procera (Nobel Biocare, Fairlawn, NJ)	600	Low
Leucite-reinforced ceramics	Empress I (Ivoclar-Vivadent, Amherst, NY)	180	Moderate
	Cerpress SL (Leach & Dillon, Cranston, RI)	180	Variable
Feldspathic ceramics	Creation (Jensen Industries, New Haven, CT)	90	High
Synthetic low-fusing quartz glass-ceramics	HeraCeram (Heraeus-Kulzer-Jelenko, Armonk, NY)	120	High

light). Value is the only tangible parameter that can be addressed; however, it is related to opacity/translucency. Certain materials are higher in translucency (eg, synthetic ceramics) while others are higher in opacity (eg, zirconia and alumina); therefore identification of the material's inherent qualities is imperative when quantifying shade (Table 2-3).

It is important to note that although the correct restorative material and shade may be selected, there is still the possibility for error due to inconsistencies and variations in the materials, for which it is difficult to control.[16–22] More-

Restorative Materials Selection

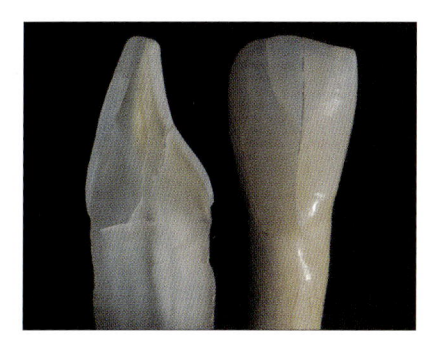

Fig 2-50
Natural extracted teeth under natural daylight conditions.

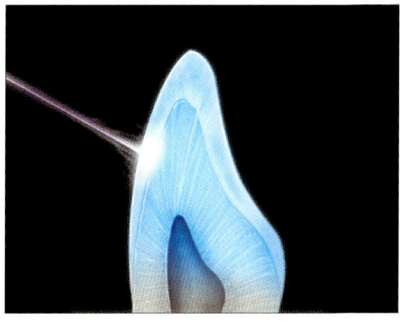

Fig 2-51
Illustration showing how ultraviolet light interacts with the cells of the dentinal layer, which emit reflected light. This phenomenon is known as *fluorescence*.

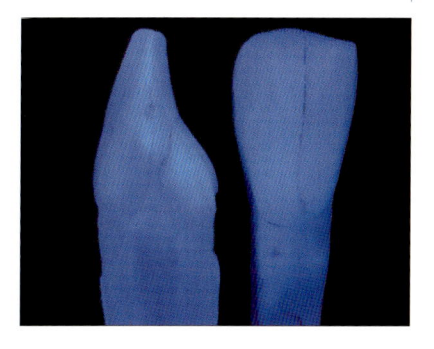

Fig 2-52
The teeth shown in Fig 2-50 under ultraviolet light. Note the greater fluorescence of the dentinal layer compared with the enamel layer.

over, improperly prepared teeth, eg, preparations with incorrect reduction, may contribute to an inaccurate shade match. However, if the protocol recommended in chapter 5 is followed, mistakes resulting from these issues should be discovered in the laboratory during shade verification and corrected before the restoration is returned for clinical try-in.

The optical triad: Fluorescence, opalescence, and translucency

For clinicians who practice esthetic restorative dentistry, particularly in the field of ceramics, fluorescence is an important physical property. By their very nature, teeth (more specifically, dentin) are fluorescent because they emit visible light when exposed to ultraviolet light (Figs 2-50 to 2-52). Porcelain consists of agents that cause the restoration to become fluorescent. Fluorescence adds to the natural look of a restoration and minimizes the metameric effect.

Opalescence is the ability of a translucent material to appear blue in reflected light and red-orange in transmitted light. The opalescent effect is based on the behavior of translucency of natural teeth. Under direct illumination, the shorter wavelengths of the visible spectrum (ie, blue wavelengths) are reflected from the fine particles of natural enamel and dental porcelain, giving the white tooth color a bluish appearance, while the longer wavelengths (ie, red-orange wavelengths) are absorbed (Fig 2-53). In transillumination, however, light penetrating through a natural tooth appears orange since the longer wavelengths

2 Elements Affecting Color

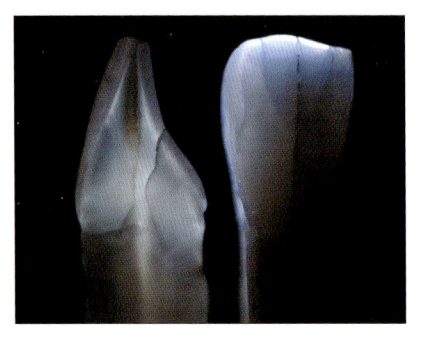

Fig 2-53
A blue opalescent effect on the teeth shown in Figs 2-50 and 2-52, caused by the reflection and transmission of blue wavelengths of light.

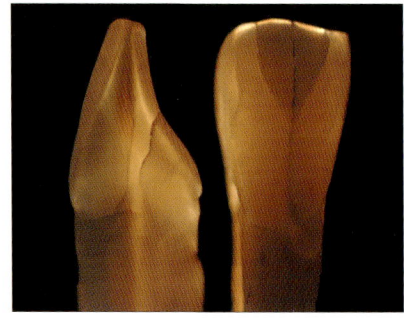

Fig 2-54
An orange opalescent effect on the teeth shown in Figs 2-50, 2-52, and 2-53, caused by the transmission and reflection of red-yellow (orange) wavelengths and the absorption of blue wavelengths.

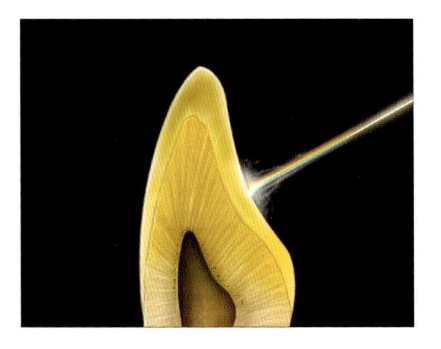

Fig 2-55
Illustration of the transmission of the longer orange wavelengths of light through the dentinal and enamel layers.

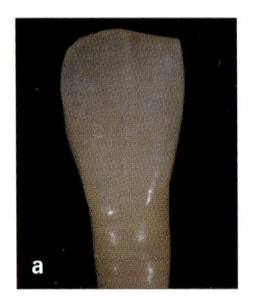

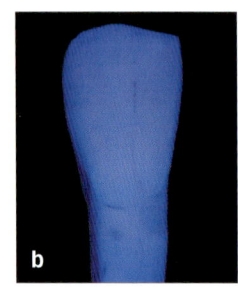

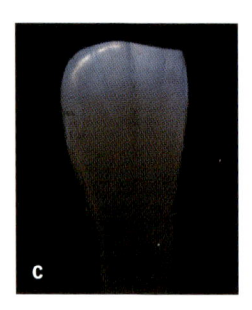

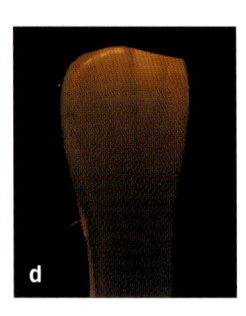

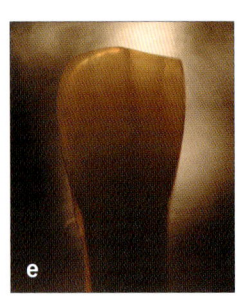

Fig 2-56
In vitro examples of light effects exhibited by a natural tooth. Natural light effects (a), fluorescence (b), opalescence (blue [c] and orange [d]), and translucency (e) are shown.

are reflected at the surface and, conversely, the shorter, blue wavelengths are absorbed (Figs 2-54 and 2-55). This effect, known in optical physics as the *Tyndall effect*, is called *opalescence of natural teeth*. Both opalescence and fluorescence are responsible for the intrinsic brilliance of natural teeth that clinicians and ceramists try to imitate when fabricating artificial restorations.[23] Likewise, depth of vitality is conveyed through translucency (Fig 2-56).

It is essential to avoid excessive opacity, which results in a lifeless-looking restoration, as well as excessive translucency, which results in a restoration that looks too gray and dark.

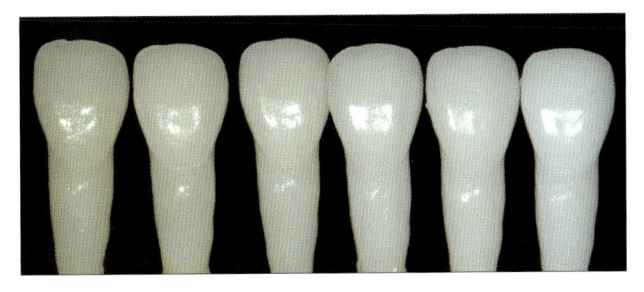

Fig 2-57
Fabricated ceramic teeth with a progression from shade B1 (Vitapan) *(far left)* to bleached shade 010 (Ivoclar) *(far right)*. (Courtesy of J. Kim, CDT.)

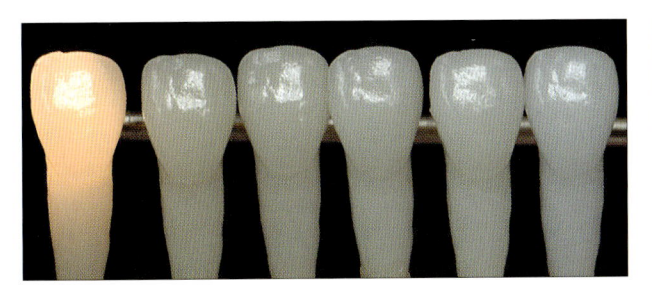

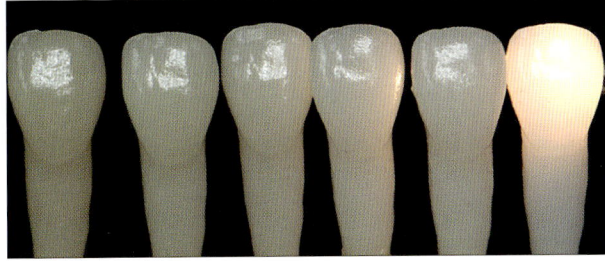

Figs 2-58 and 2-59
Light transillumination of B1 shade (Fig 2-58) and bleached shade 010 (Fig 2-59) shows that both shades allow the same amount of light transmission. Therefore, fabricated teeth can be white and bright while maintaining a high level of translucency. (Courtesy of J. Kim, CDT.)

Bleaching

Most people say they want *white* teeth. However, the color white is scientifically described as being completely reflective of all visible wavelengths of light, which implies an opacity that is undesirable in the dentition. In the context of esthetic dentistry, *white* as an ideal tooth color refers to the lightness or translucency of a tooth or restoration. When teeth are bleached, the relative lightness (value) of the teeth is increased, making them appear whiter. Therefore, bleaching does not necessarily involve making the teeth more opaque and reflective; rather, intrinsic colored pigments are removed, allowing a tooth to become whiter yet remain highly translucent (Figs 2-57 to 2-59). Usually, bleaching is performed through the application of a gel containing oxidants (eg, carbamide-peroxide). Oxygen radicals released from the gel penetrate the enamel and oxidize many of the dark colorants in the dentinal layer that may be of intrinsic or extrinsic origin. The structure of teeth remains the same, while the value of the teeth increases.

Conclusions

There are several factors that can influence the dental professional's color assessment. When using traditional shade-matching techniques, there are several variables that the dental professional should consider. For example, changes in operatory lighting, fatigued eyes, and various contrast effects can create optical illusions. Additionally, the side effects associated with the use of oral contraceptives are a problem for female practitioners, and the high incidence of color blindness among US males is of equal concern. Although no dental practitioner can read color perfectly, and no dental operatory is free from problems, a thorough understanding of the potential factors affecting color perception allows the dental professional to compensate for them as required to achieve the most accurate shade match possible.

Summary

- Lighting plays a critical role in shade matching. Color can appear different under operatory lighting than it does in natural light. The dental professional should be prepared to compensate for this phenomenon.
- Various contrast effects (value, hue, chroma, areal, spatial, and successive) can create optical illusions that interfere with accurate color evaluation. However, in some cases, effects such as hue contrast can be used to improve color perception.
- An individual's overall health is connected to the health of the eyes, which can greatly affect the observer's color perception.
- As dental professionals age, their color perception is greatly affected.
- The selection of restorative materials plays a pivotal role in the determination of shade.

References

1. Sim CP, Yap AU, Teo J. Color perception among different dental personnel. Oper Dent 2001;26:435–439.
2. Carsten D. Successful shade matching—What does it take? Compend Contin Educ Dent 2003;24:175–178,180,182.
3. Lamb T, Bourriau J (eds). Colour: Art and Science. Cambridge, UK: Cambridge University Press, 1995.
4. Commission Internationale de l'Eclairage. Colorimetry, Official Recommendations of the International Commission on Illumination [Publication CIE No. 15 (E-1.3.1)]. Paris: Bureau Central de la CIE, 1971.
5. Bunting F. The ColorShop Color Primer. Available at: http://www.xrite.com/documents/mktg/ColorPrimer.pdf. Accessed 18 September 2003.
6. Chu SJ. Color. In: Gürel G (ed). The Science and Art of Porcelain Laminate Veneers. Chicago: Quintessence, 2003:158–206.
7. Sproull RC. Color matching in dentistry, part I. The three-dimensional nature of color. J Prosthet Dent 1973;29:416–424.
8. Albers J. Interaction of Color. New Haven, CT: Yale University Press, 1971.
9. Wasson W, Schuman N. Color vision and dentistry. Quintessence Int 1992;23:349–353.
10. Quackenbush TR. Relearning to See. Berkeley, CA: North Atlantic Books, 1997.
11. Rosenthal O, Phillips R. Coping with Color-Blindness. New York: Avery, 1997.
12. The Schepens Eye Research Institute website. Available at http://www.eri.harvard.edu. Accessed 6 October 2003.
13. Age-Related Eye Disease Study Research Group. A randomized, placebo-controlled, clinical trial of high-dose supplementation with vitamins C and E, beta carotene, and zinc for age-related macular degeneration and vision loss: AREDS report no. 8. Arch Ophthalmol 2001; 119:1417–1436.
14. Gimbel T. Healing with Color and Light. New York: Simon and Schuster, 1994.
15. Fraunfelder FT. Drug-Induced Ocular Side Effects. Philadelphia: Williams & Wilkins, 1996.
16. Reich S, Hornberger H. The effect of multicolored machinable ceramics on the esthetics of all-ceramic crowns. J Prosthet Dent 2002;88:44–49.
17. Wee AG, Monaghan P, Johnston WM. Variation in color between intended matched shade and fabricated shade of dental porcelain. J Prosthet Dent 2002;87:657–666.
18. Lichter JA, Solomowitz BH, Sher M. Shade selection. Communicating with the laboratory technician. N Y State Dent J 2000;66(5):42–46.
19. Geary JL, Kinirons MJ. Colour perception of laboratory-fired samples of body-coloured ceramic. J Dent 1999;27:145–148.
20. Rosenstiel SF, Porter SS, Johnston WM. Colour measurements of all ceramic crown systems. J Oral Rehabil 1989;16:491–501.
21. Ecker GA, Moser JB. Visual and instrumental discrimination steps between two adjacent porcelain shades. J Prosthet Dent 1987;58:286–291.
22. Seghi RR, Johnston WM, O'Brien WJ. Spectrophotometric analysis of color differences between porcelain systems. J Prosthet Dent 1986;56:35–40.
23. Leinfelder K. Porcelain esthetics for the 21st century. J Am Dent Assoc 2000;131(suppl): 47S–51S.

3 Conventional Shade Matching

In this chapter:
- Step-by-step process
- Shade guide systems
- Recommended protocol
- Special considerations for direct composites

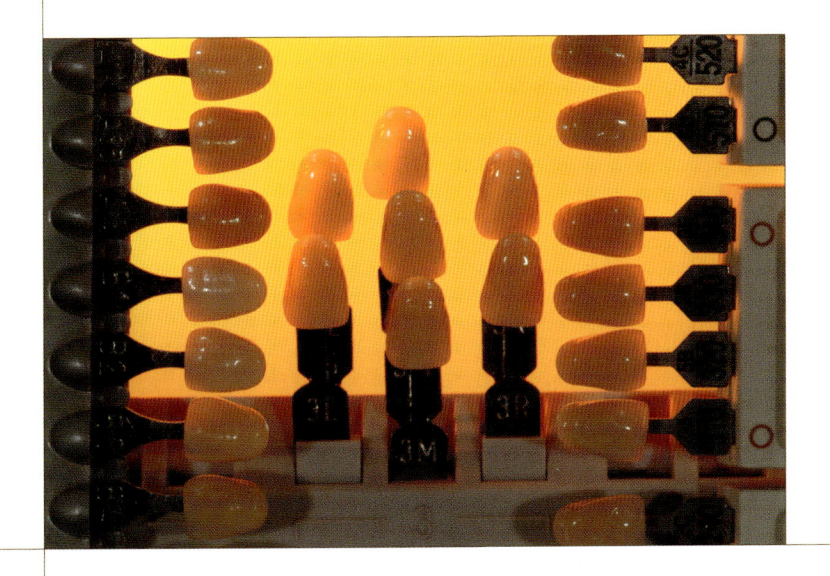

3 Conventional Shade Matching

For nearly a century, dental professionals have relied on shade tabs for an "accurate" shade match. Unfortunately, this conventional form of shade taking is oversimplified, and relying on it alone almost guarantees an esthetic mismatch. There is too much subjectivity and too little offered in terms of a legitimate standard. However, shade tabs are useful as visual guides if not as definitive answers; therefore, the following conventional method does have its merits, particularly when used in conjunction with technology-based shade matching (see chapter 5).

Step-by-Step Process

The conventional shade-matching process can be divided into five distinct steps: analysis, communication, interpretation, fabrication, and verification. Each of these steps involves a certain amount of subjective evaluation.

Analysis

Shade analysis is a careful, time-consuming process. It should be carried out under color-corrected lighting, and, ideally, shades also should be checked in natural light. Moreover, determining one base shade is not sufficient to obtain an esthetic shade match. The clinician must match each of three sections of the tooth: gingival, body, and incisal (Fig 3-1).

The first step in analysis is to determine whether the tooth is high in opacity or translucency (Figs 3-2 and 3-3). This information will aid in the material selection process. Then, the clinician must find the brightness, or value, for each section of the tooth. Value control is critical because, as discussed in chapter 2, value determination directly affects the materials and type of restoration to be used, which correlate to the required tooth preparation design. Unfortunately, shade tabs are not representative of the value of real teeth, which is why relying on shade tab assessment alone can be problematic.[1]

Next, the chroma, or saturation of tooth color, must be evaluated. An example of high chroma is the deep orange quality often found in the teeth of elderly patients (Fig 3-4).

Step-by-Step Process

Fig 3-1
The polychromatic effects of teeth should be noted and identified with shade tabs for each of the three distinct color zones within a tooth: gingival (G), body (B), and incisal (I).

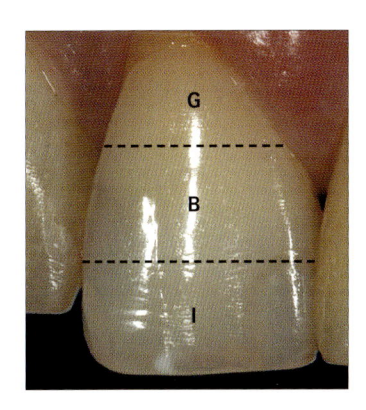

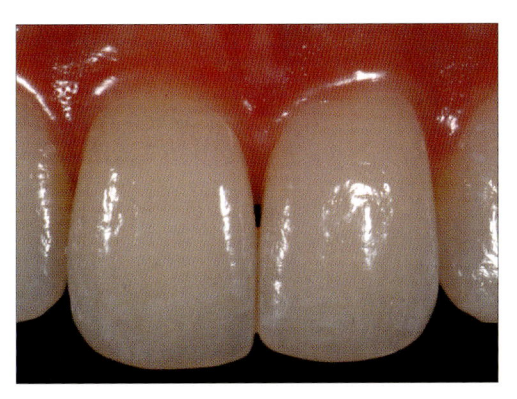

Fig 3-2
Clinical example of maxillary central incisors that are somewhat higher in opacity and lower in translucency.

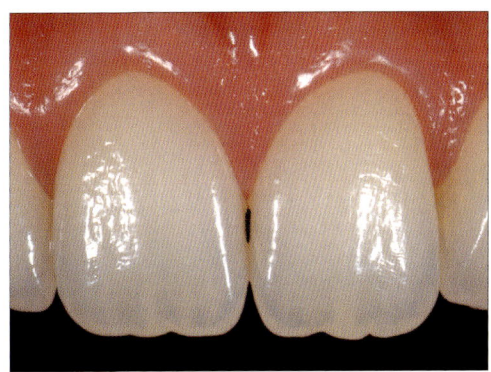

Fig 3-3
Clinical example of maxillary central incisors that are relatively lower in opacity and higher in translucency.

Fig 3-4
Clinical example of an elderly patient's maxillary central incisors with highly chromatic amber translucency. As the enamel layer becomes thinner with age, the more chromatic dentinal color shows through the tooth, creating a warm, amber color.

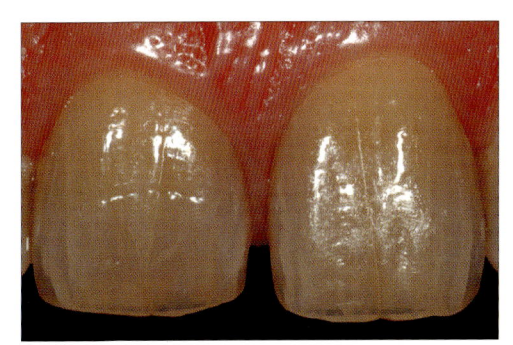

Recently bleached teeth are high in value and low in chroma. A very white tooth can sometimes be the most difficult to match because it does not match most traditional shade guides, and bleached shade tabs are limited in their number and scope. To match a bleached tooth, the clinician should analyze the color under various lighting conditions to ensure the accuracy of the shade.

3 CONVENTIONAL SHADE MATCHING

Fig 3-5
Pretreatment clinical image of a patient with "Hollywood" expectations. These patients are vocal about treatment expectations and seek a whiter, straighter appearance of their restorations.

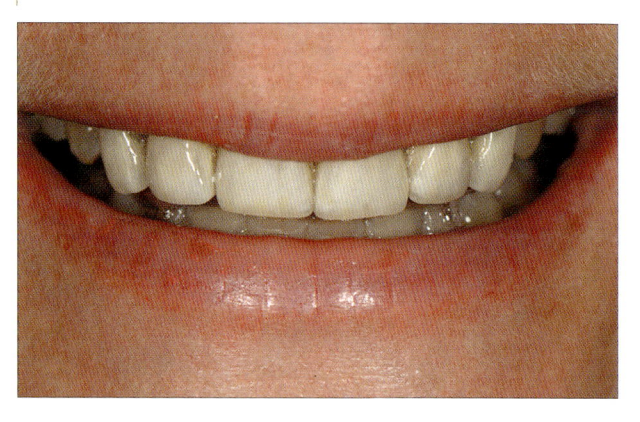

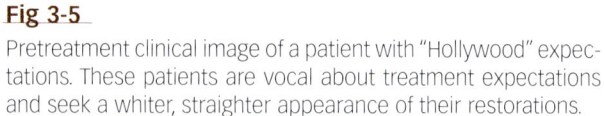

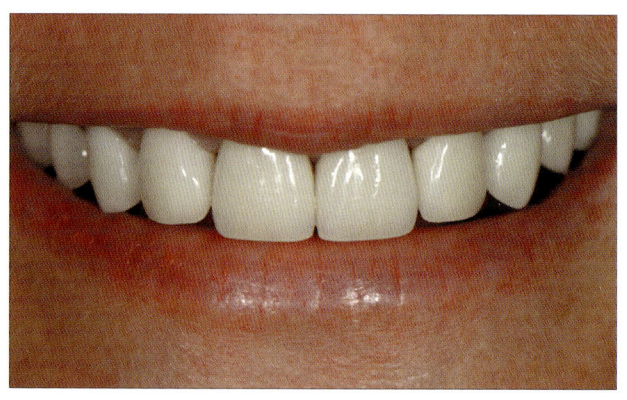

Fig 3-6
Patient shown in Fig 3-5 following treatment.

It is also important during shade analysis to determine the patient's expectations for treatment. Generally, patient expectations fall into one of three categories:

- *Hollywood.* White and straight restorations. These patients are generally very concerned and vocal (Figs 3-5 and 3-6).
- *Alfred E. Newman.* Restorative design according to the clinician's expertise. The vast majority of patients fall into this category, although most will lean toward one of the other two categories (Figs 3-7 and 3-8).
- *Naturalist.* Restorations that look natural and blend in completely with the rest of the dentition. These patients are often the most difficult to treat because they may have numerous craze lines, wear facets, diastemas, strange rotations, and specific contours that will have to be matched (Figs 3-9 to 3-12).

Shade analysis is a demanding process; however, it should be performed as expediently as possible. If analysis takes too long, the clinician's eyes will become increasingly fatigued, making it difficult, if not impossible, to take an accurate shade.

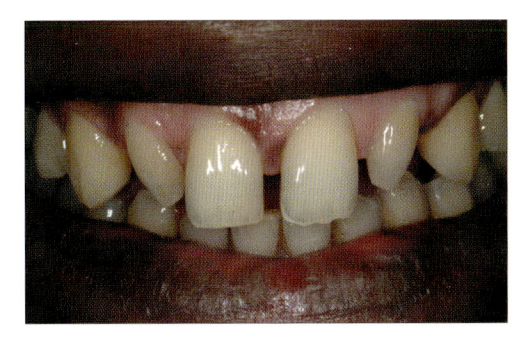

Step-by-Step Process

Fig 3-7
Pretreatment clinical image of a patient with "Alfred E. Newman" expectations. These patients are easier to treat because they are more accepting of what the clinician prescribes. They can accept a straight and white or a clean and natural appearance.

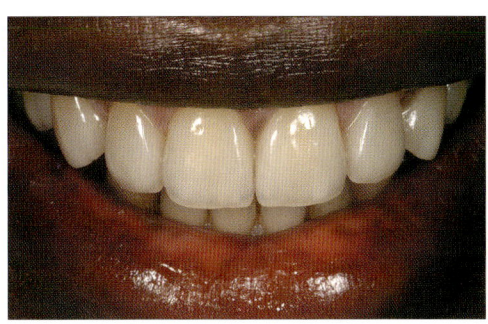

Fig 3-8
Patient shown in Fig 3-7 following treatment.

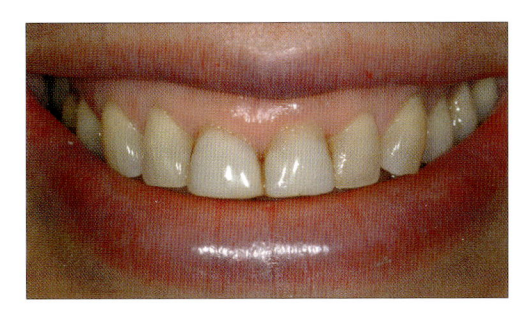

Fig 3-9
Pretreatment clinical image of a patient with "naturalist" expectations. These patients can be the most demanding because they seek a realistic esthetic restorative effect.

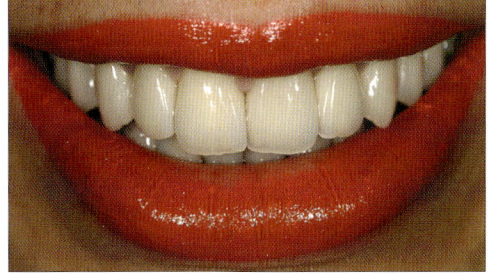

Fig 3-10
Patient shown in Fig 3-9 following treatment. This patient is accepting of incisal irregularities, mamelon ceramic incisal effects, and slight rotations of the maxillary incisors.

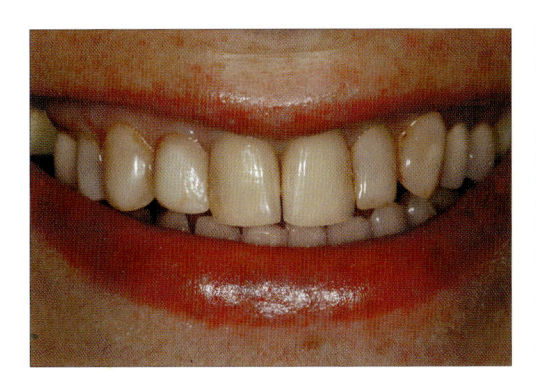

Fig 3-11
Pretreatment clinical image of a patient with "naturalist" expectations.

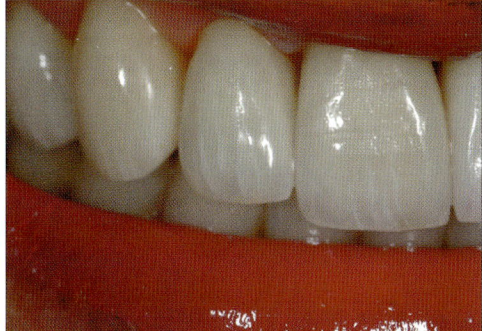

Fig 3-12
Patient shown in Fig 3-11 following treatment. This patient is accepting of internal characterization effects (multiple white craze lines) of the ceramic laminate veneer restorations.

3 Conventional Shade Matching

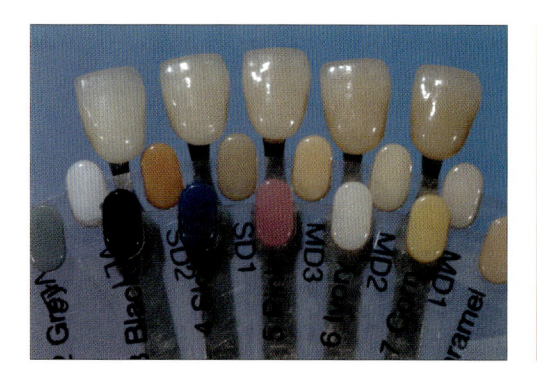

Fig 3-13
The conversion of shade tab information into ceramic effect powders is vital to color communication.

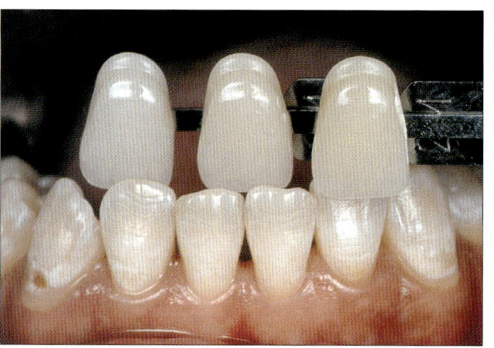

Fig 3-14
An aggregate in vivo photograph of shade tabs for each section of the tooth (gingival, body, and incisal). This visual communication tool helps the technician evaluate value and chroma.

Communication

In the conventional shade-matching system, while the clinician is working solely with shade tabs, the lab technician must take the basic information about value and chroma provided by the shade tabs and apply that information to the ceramic system and effect powders being used (Fig 3-13). That is why effective communication between the lab technician and the clinician is critical to achieving a successful shade match. Color is a unique language spoken by the clinician and the lab technician. Acronyms abound, and a firm grasp of the language is a prerequisite to effective communication between the clinician and the lab technician. The situation is further complicated when different materials and labs are used.

Each porcelain system has its own color-matching system and nomenclature. Some labs and technicians may fear switching materials because of a lack of confidence not in the material, but rather in their shade-matching ability using the "color language" of a different porcelain system. It is best to partner with a lab that is skilled in shade matching using several varieties of materials.

It is suggested that the clinician send photographs along with the shade tabs as reference. Photography is a great means of communication between the clinician and the lab technician and adds credibility to the shade tab selection. Once the gingival, body, and incisal shade tabs are selected, photographs of each of the tabs should be taken next to the tooth to be matched, together with an aggregate photograph of all three tabs near the dentition (Fig 3-14). It also makes

Step-by-Step Process

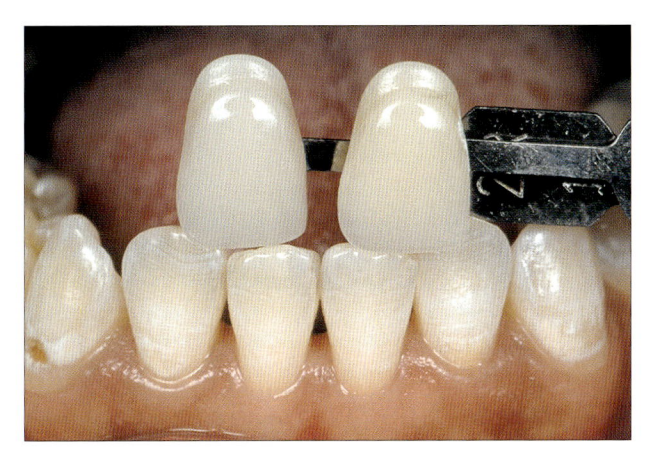

Fig 3-15
Reference photograph captured using a neutral flash (color temperature of 5,500 K).

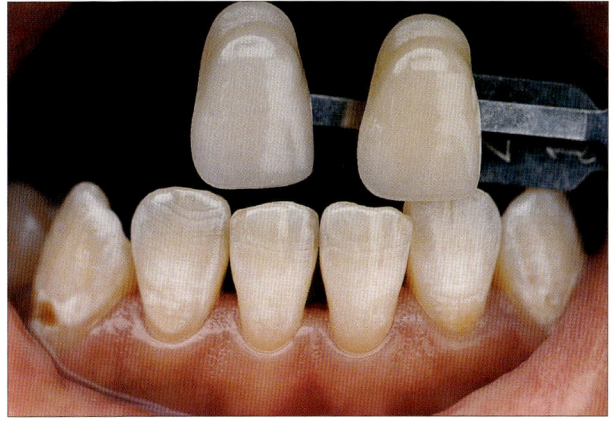

Fig 3-16
Teeth and shade tabs shown in Fig 3-15 captured using a flash with a color temperature of 6,500 K. Note how the color of the photograph changes. This can negatively influence color interpretation by the technician.

sense to photograph the matched tooth next to the two extreme shades (one lighter than the perceived shade and one darker); this allows the lab technician to get a concrete sense of the shade and value variation. Finally, photographs should be taken of the patient's face and full smile to allow the technician to envision how the restoration will fit into the patient's overall appearance.

When taking reference photographs to send to a lab, it is important to remember that a different flash on the camera changes the appearance of the teeth and shade tabs because of the variation in color temperature (Figs 3-15 and 3-16). Therefore, selecting the correct color temperature of the flash (5,500 K) is critical to capturing unbiased shade information in a photograph.

The detailed communication of color is critical to the successful delivery of esthetically pleasing restorations. In conventional shade matching, a majority of the color determination is performed visually by both the clinician and the lab technician. This subjectivity involved in assessing color is one of the most difficult barriers to accurate communication between the clinician and technician.[2]

3 Conventional Shade Matching

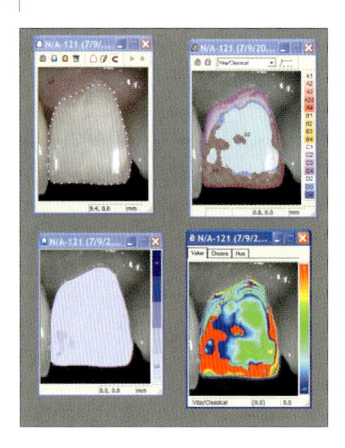

Fig 3-17
Preoperative ShadeScan (Cynovad, Montreal, Canada) of the maxillary left central incisor to be matched. The base shade is Vita D2.

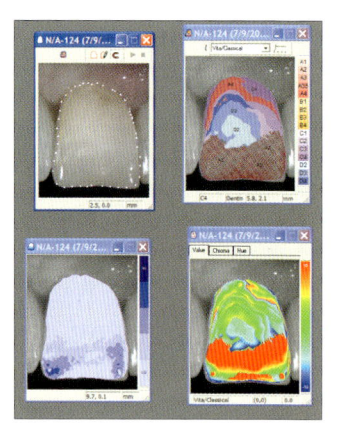

Fig 3-18
ShadeScan of the restoration fabricated for the maxillary right central incisor showing a similar base shade of Vita D2.

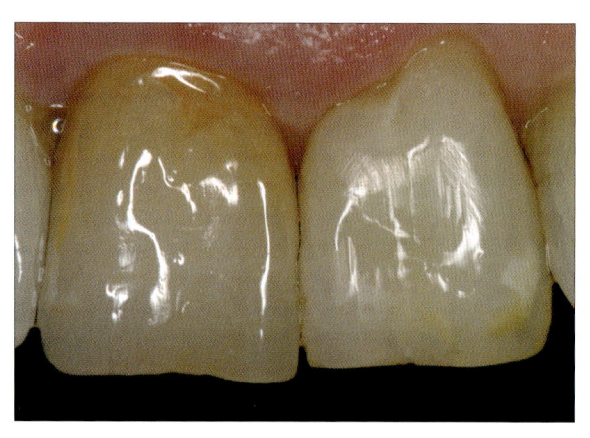

Fig 3-19
Clinical photograph showing the restoration in place. It does not appear to be a close match because its surface texture and luster are wrong, which dramatically influences the surface reflectance and therefore the perceived shade.

Interpretation

The interpretation process involves looking at the restoration against a gray background (18% reflectance), then creating a color map for fabricating the restoration. Although lab technicians are skilled in these procedures, even an expert cannot create a successful match when provided with bad data. Therefore, it is the job of the clinician to ensure that the information provided to the technician is as accurate as possible.

Fabrication

In order to fabricate a highly esthetic, accurate restoration, the lab technician must study the unique characteristics of the tooth in the clinical close-up photograph. The fabrication process is extremely sensitive. Even if the color is matched accurately, surface characteristics such as glaze, texture, and luster can alter the color of the restoration, possibly causing an apparent mismatch (Figs 3-17 to 3-19). This is because, as discussed in chapter 1, what the eye perceives as color is actually the reflection of light.

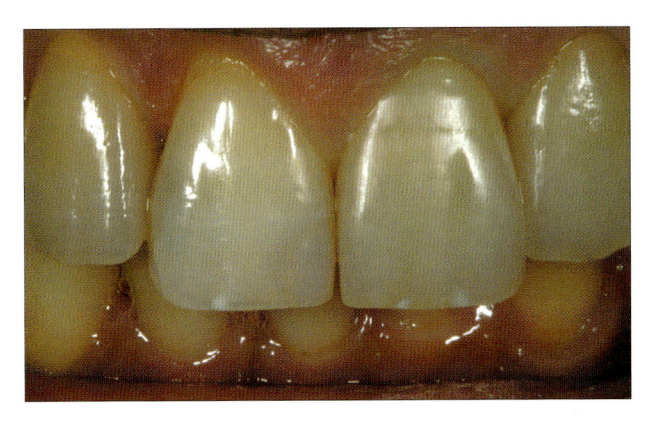

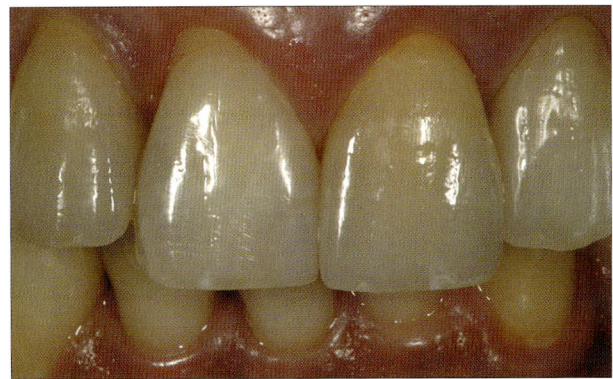

Figs 3-20 and 3-21
Visual shade verification can be performed in an instant. Either the restoration matches (Fig 3-20) or it doesn't (Fig 3-21).

It is important to discuss with the lab technician which materials will work best for a given case. Even within the genre of porcelain materials, there are differences in opacity and translucency. For instance, zirconium-based materials are the least translucent; fully synthetic ceramics are the most translucent.

Verification

With a conventional approach, the best way to verify a restoration is simply to look at it. It is immediately clear if the tooth shade or value is off (Figs 3-20 and 3-21).

Shade Guide Systems

Because of their inherent subjectivity, inconsistencies have been documented in conventional shade guide systems. For example, the Vita Classical shade guide (Vita, Bad Sackingen, Germany) is too low in chroma and too high in value when compared to extracted tooth samples,[1,3,4] and the Vita Lumin A3 shade tabs may vary within and among several guides used by the same manufacturer. The Vita Classical, Chromascop (Ivoclar-Vivadent, Amherst, NY), and Vitapan 3D-Master (Vita) are currently the most popular shade guides.[5]

3 Conventional Shade Matching

Vita Classical

In the Vita Classical shade guide, hue is categorized by letters:

- A = Orange
- B = Yellow
- C = Yellow/Gray
- D = Orange/Gray (Brown)

Chroma and value are communicated by a system of numbers:

- 1 = Least chromatic, highest value
- 4 = Most chromatic, lowest value

Chromascop

The Chromascop system uses a numbering system to identify the shade:

- 100 = White
- 200 = Yellow
- 300 = Orange
- 400 = Gray
- 500 = Brown

Chroma and value are communicated by another system of numbers:

- 10 = Least chromatic, highest value
- 40 = Most chromatic, lowest value

Vitapan 3D-Master

The Vitapan 3D-Master is a unique departure from the conventional lettering/numbering categorization systems. This product, created based on research by some of the industry's leading authorities on color,[4,6] has improved conventional shade matching by removing some of the subjectivity from shade tab–based color assessment. Using this system, shade selection is a logical progression of three simplified steps, enabling the clinician to find the desired shade quickly.

Shade Guide Systems

Fig 3-22 With lighter shades, hue is difficult to discern because chroma is so low. It is difficult to determine which shade tab is a B1 *(left)* and which is an A1 *(right)*.

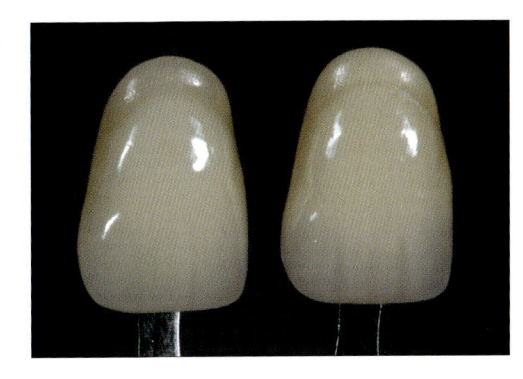

1. *Value (lightness) determination.* The dental professional selects the value level (from 1 to 5, with 1 being the lightest [high value] and 5 being the darkest [low value]) that is closest to the value of the tooth to be matched, then takes the medium (M) shade sample from the selected value group.
2. *Chroma determination.* The clinician selects the color sample from the M group with the chroma level (from 1 to 3, with 1 being the least chromatic and 3 being the most chromatic) that is closest to that of the tooth to be matched.
3. *Hue determination.* The clinician checks whether the natural tooth displays a more yellowish (L) or more reddish (R) shade than the color sample of the M group selected in the second step. Now the best-matching shade sample can be determined and the information recorded in the color communication form.

Value-based versus hue-based shade guides

Value-based shade guides are a more accurate means of shade selection. Recently, the Vita Classical shade guide has been rearranged according to a value-based ordering system (B1, A1, A2, D2, B2, C1, C2, D4, D3, A3, B3, A3.5, B4, C3, A4, C4). The human eye is more sensitive to changes in value rather than subtle changes in hue. This is especially true with bleached shades, which, as previously noted, are some of the most difficult shades to match. When examining a B1 versus an A1 shade tab, it is difficult to assess which tab contains more yellow and which contains more orange (Fig 3-22).

In most cases, if value and chroma are correct, the restoration will be clinically acceptable, even if the hue is slightly off.

3 Conventional Shade Matching

Recommended Protocol (Figs 3-23 to 3-50)

1. The patient removes any lipstick or other makeup that could affect shade matching. If the patient is wearing bright clothing, it is prudent to cover the patient with a neutral-colored bib (Figs 3-23 to 3-26).
2. The existing tooth structure on which the restoration will be fabricated is evaluated (eg, whether it is vital or discolored by previous endodontic work or metal restorations). This will influence tooth preparation design and material selection (Figs 3-27 and 3-28).
3. The translucency and opacity of the patient's natural teeth are determined. This will help in the material selection process (Figs 3-29 to 3-31).
4. The shade selection is made at the beginning of the appointment, before the eyes become too fatigued. It is important not to view the comparison for more than 7 seconds at a time to avoid fatiguing the cones of the retina. Also, it is important to determine the shade when the teeth are most hydrated—teeth dry out during the preparation and impression-making procedures.
5. A variety of shade tabs are used to analyze the opposing dentition's value in the gingival, body, and incisal areas. Value is analyzed first, followed by chroma, then hue (Figs 3-32 and 3-33).
6. Once an ideal match has been selected, extreme shade tabs (light and dark) are photographed next to the teeth to be matched (Fig 3-34).
7. The full smile is photographed (Fig 3-35).
8. Provisional restorations are fabricated to restore proper tissue health, esthetics, tooth contours, and occlusion and to provide information to the technician regarding incisal length and overjet/overbite (Fig 3-36).
9. All of the information is processed and the materials sent (as hard copies or as electronic files via e-mail or on CD) to the lab technician.
10. The lab technician analyzes the information and creates a color map (Fig 3-37).
11. The lab technician fabricates the restoration and adds any details that are shown in the reference photographs (Figs 3-38 to 3-44).
12. The lab technician compares the final restoration to the reference photographs as well as the shade tabs and makes any adjustments necessary before sending it to the clinician.
13. The clinician tries in the restoration and verifies the shade match. This visual verification should be performed under several lighting conditions (eg, color-corrected light and natural daylight) to ensure the accuracy of the match. In this case, the process of analysis, communication, and fabri-

Recommended Protocol

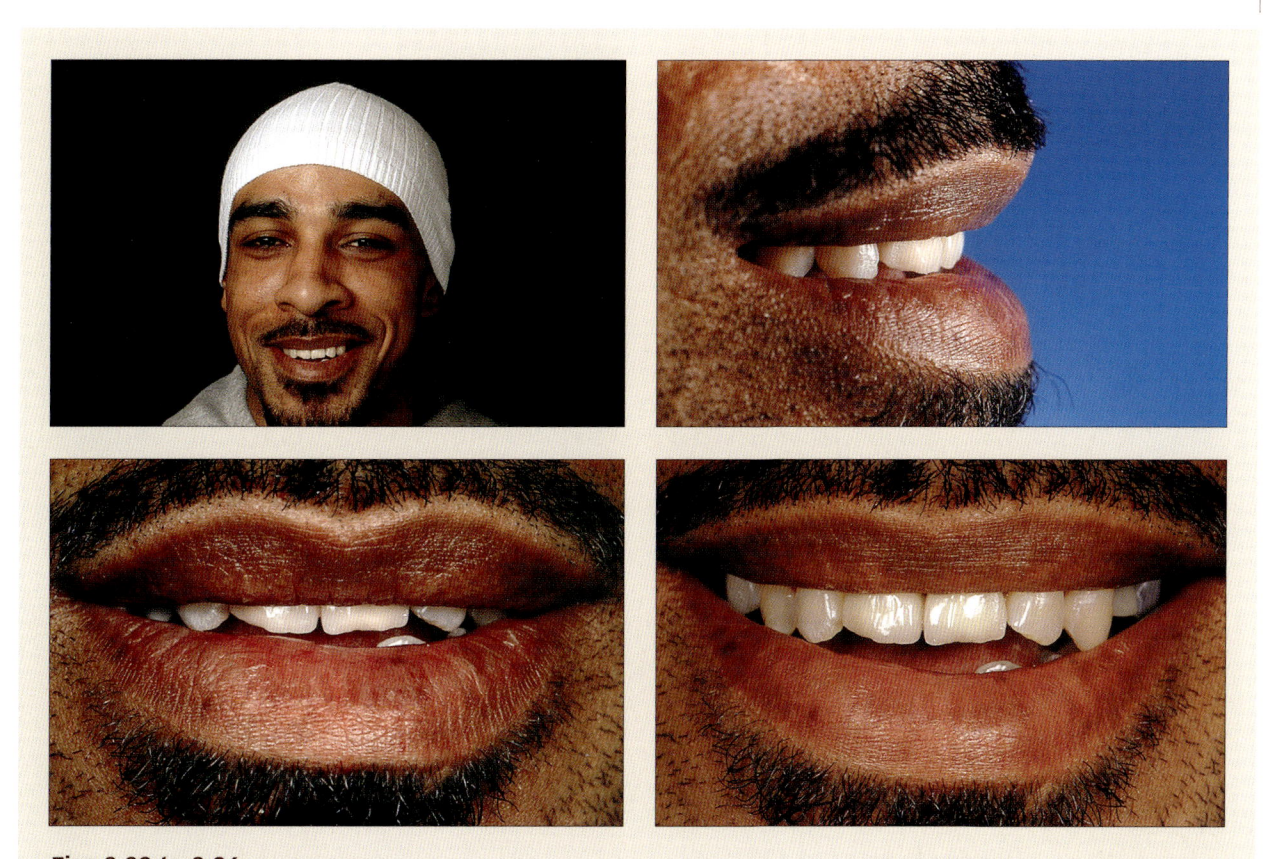

Figs 3-23 to 3-26
Preoperative clinical photographs. All surrounding distractions that could negatively affect shade matching and communication have been removed.

cation had to be repeated for three different sets of restorations before an acceptable shade match was achieved (Figs 3-45 to 3-50). Using technology-based shade-matching techniques in conjunction with this conventional protocol would improve the results (see chapter 5).

3 Conventional Shade Matching

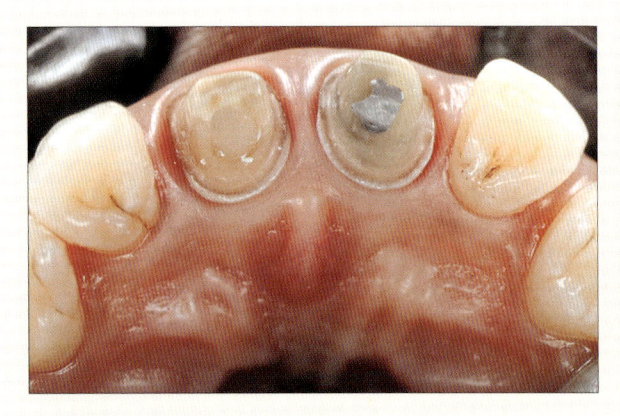

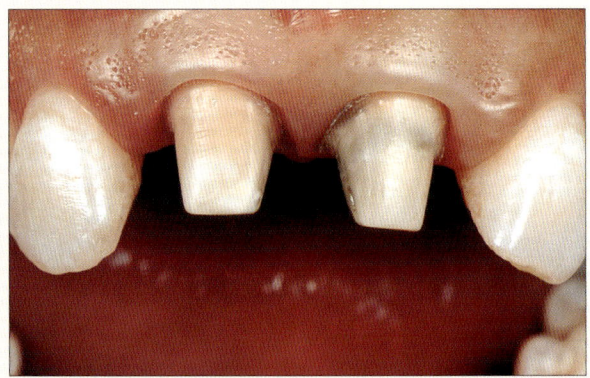

Figs 3-27 and 3-28
The maxillary central incisors are both nonvital; however, the left central incisor presents with greater discoloration as well as a non-tooth-colored core restoration (amalgam). This may impact the technical fabrication of the restorations if an all-ceramic material is chosen.

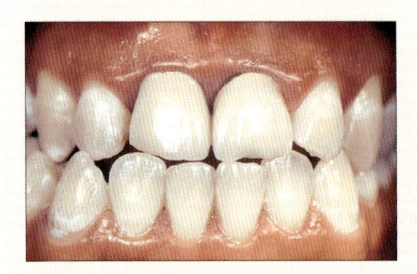

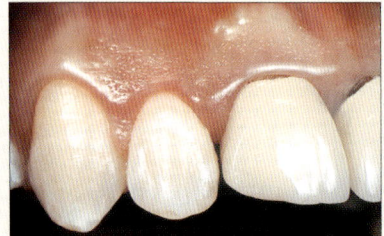

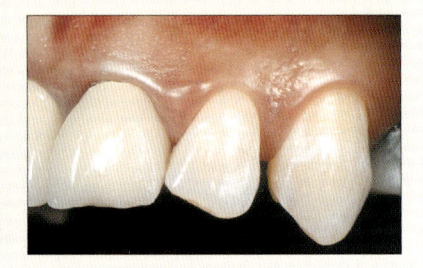

Figs 3-29 to 3-31
The relative translucency of the teeth to be matched is determined. Different views and evaluation of different teeth are helpful in assessing this parameter.

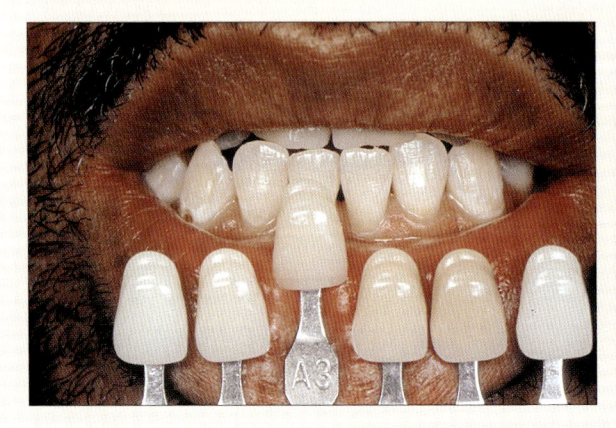

Fig 3-32
The Vita Classical shade guide is used to select the shade of the teeth in the opposing arch.

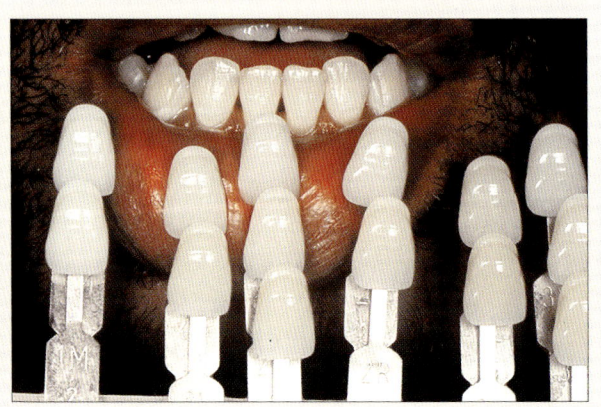

Fig 3-33
The Vitapan 3D-Master is used as a comparative analysis of shade. Using a variety of shade guides is helpful for accurate and comprehensive shade determination.

RECOMMENDED PROTOCOL

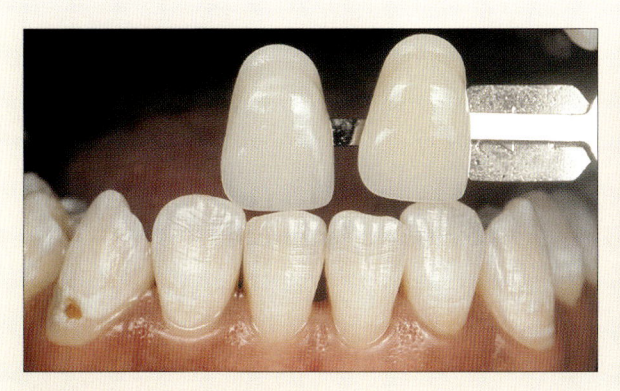

Fig 3-34
Reference photograph of extreme shade tabs (light and dark) for value determination.

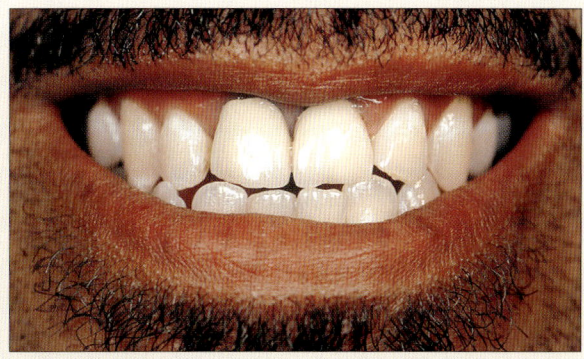

Fig 3-35
A photograph of the full smile.

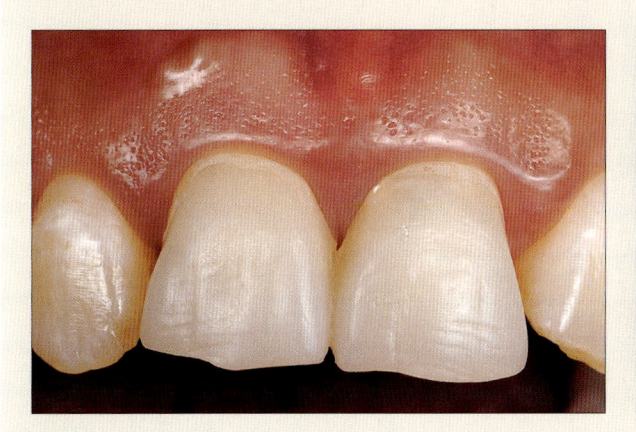

Fig 3-36
Provisional restorations in place.

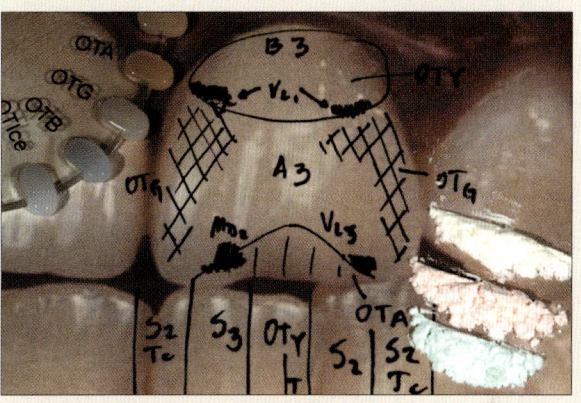

Fig 3-37
The shade information is interpreted. Effect powders are selected and a laboratory shade map is drawn in the language of the ceramic system used.

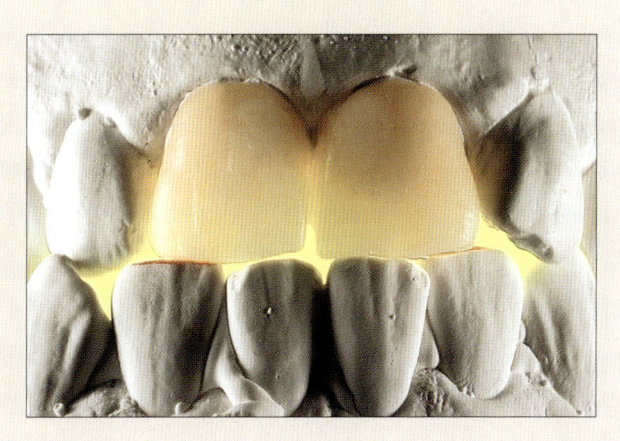

Fig 3-38
Waxup of the restorations.

65

3 Conventional Shade Matching

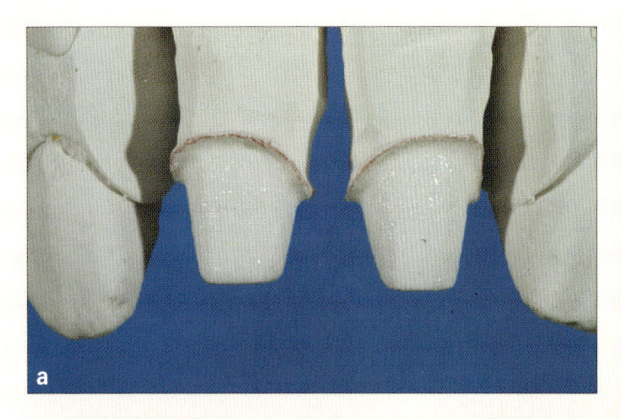

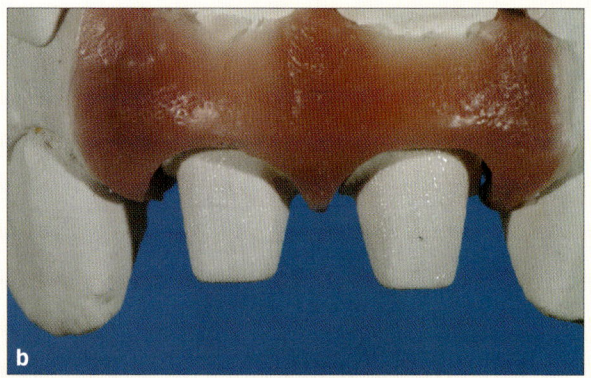

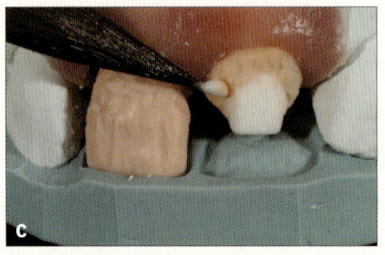

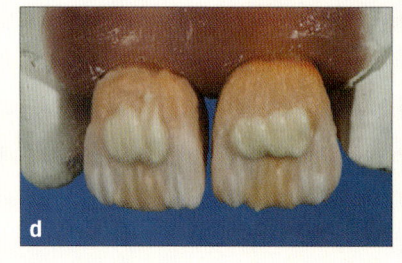

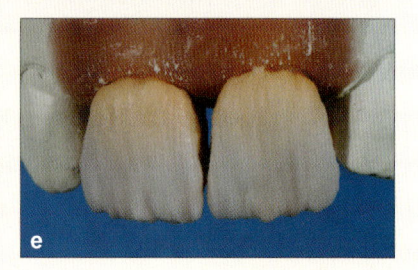

Fig 3-39
Ceramic layering of the restorations.

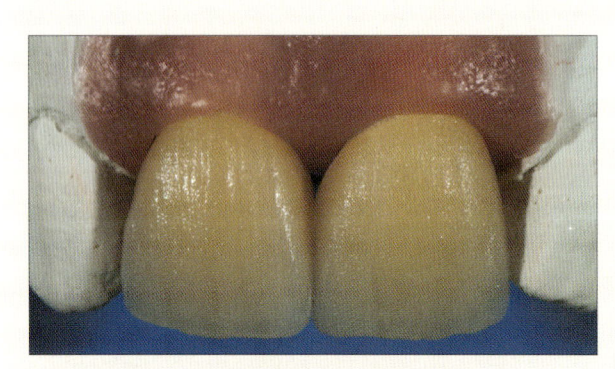

Figs 3-40 to 3-42
The restorations are finished and contoured, and surface texture is created.

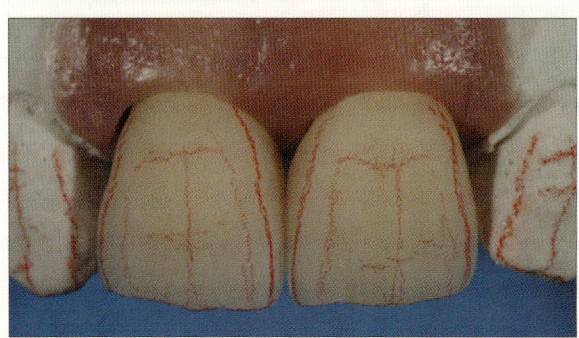

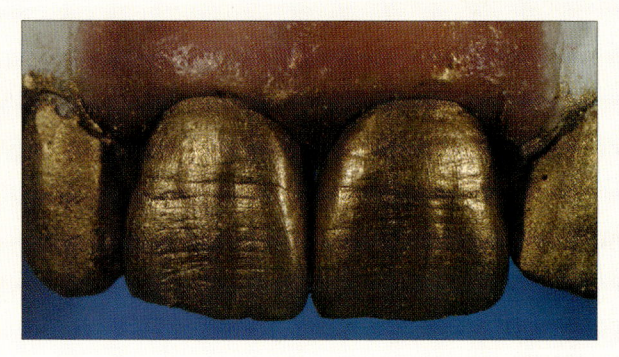

RECOMMENDED PROTOCOL

Fig 3-43
The restorations are glazed (a). Translucency (b) and fluorescence (c) are exhibited.

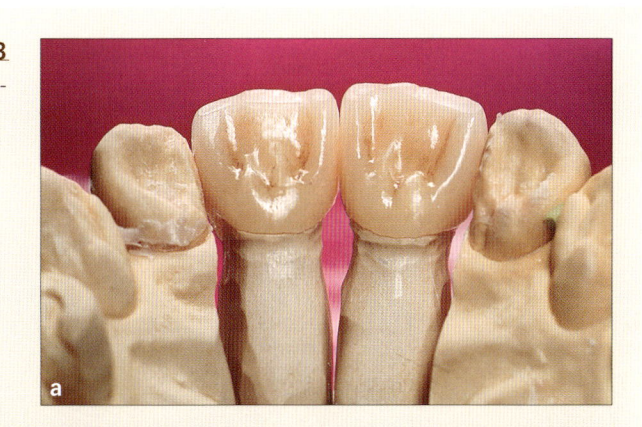

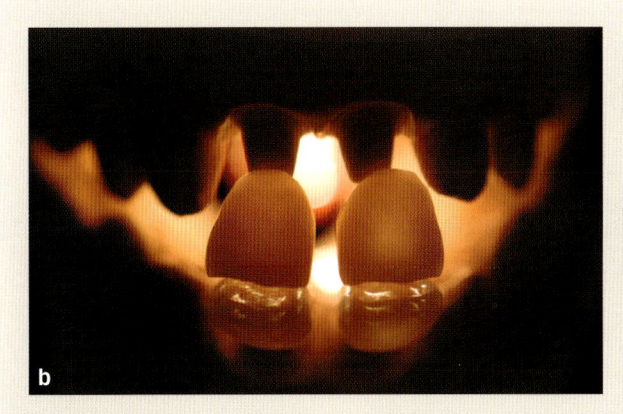

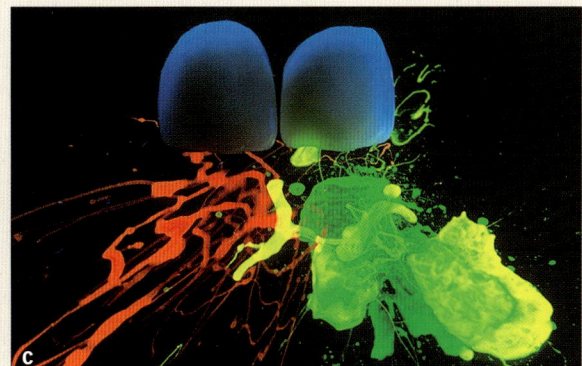

Fig 3-44
The restorations are fitted on the solid cast.

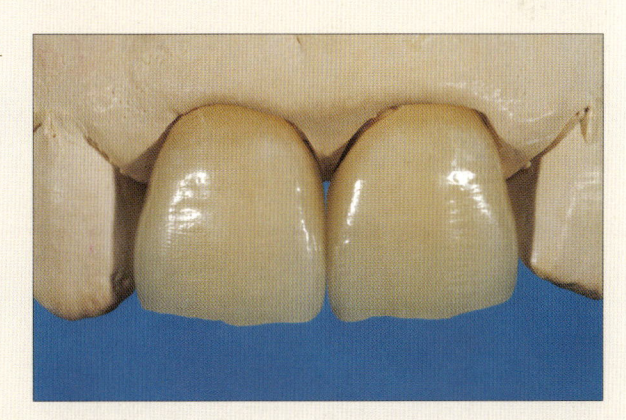

67

3 Conventional Shade Matching

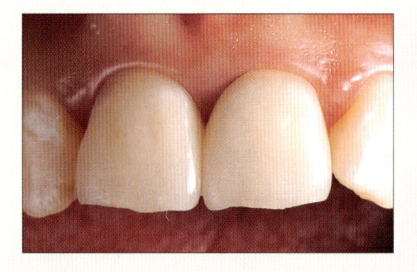

Fig 3-45
The first crowns fabricated were too opaque.

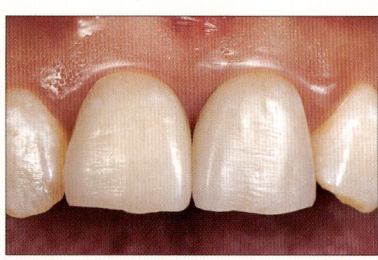

Fig 3-46
The second set of crowns was too dark.

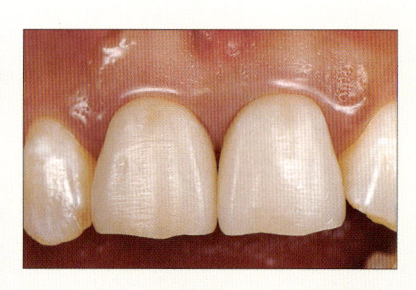

Fig 3-47
A clinically acceptable match was achieved with the third and final set of crowns.

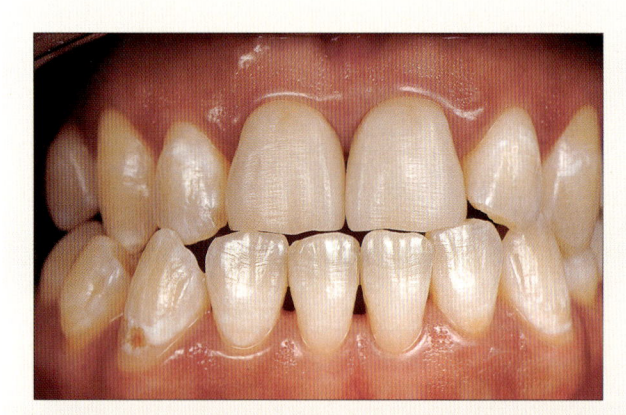

Figs 3-48 to 3-50
Postoperative clinical photographs showing the final restorations in place.

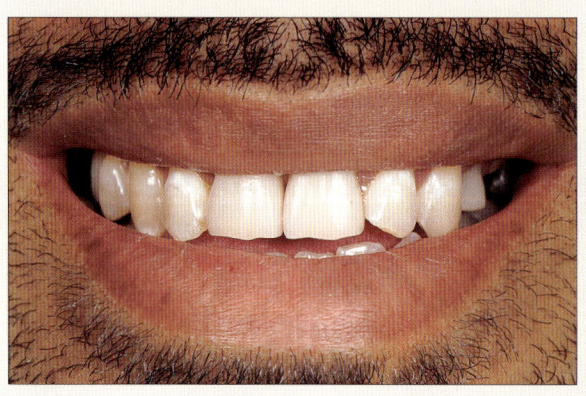

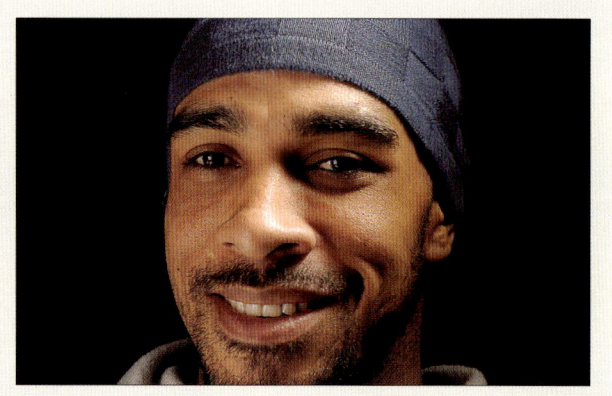

Fig 3-51 Transillumination of natural teeth, showing the enamel as a translucent shell around the colored dentin.

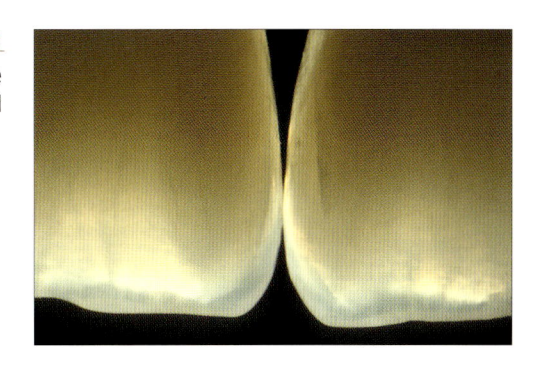

Special Considerations for Direct Composites

Though many regard ceramics as the restorative material of choice, composite materials have been gaining favor because of their excellent esthetic potential, acceptable longevity, and relatively low cost.[7,8] In addition, direct composites allow for minimally invasive preparation or require no preparation and are indicated for Class 3, 4, and 5 restorations and for esthetic correction of tooth form, dimension, and color.

Modern fabrication of composite restorations is based on the *natural layering concept*.[9,10] This approach embraces the typical optical and anatomic characteristics of natural teeth[7,9,11] and emphasizes the importance of using materials specifically designed to emulate the dentin and enamel, respectively. According to this concept, the dentin replacement materials should be characterized by:

- Single opacity
- Single hue
- Large chroma scale
- Fluorescence

The enamel replacement materials should mimic the different kinds of natural enamels, which for practical reasons are classified into three types:

- *Young enamel.* White tint, high opalescence, lower translucency
- *Adult enamel.* Neutral tint, less opalescence, intermediate translucency
- *Aged enamel.* Yellow or grayish tint, higher translucency

Of course, identification of the optical characteristics of dentin and enamel is of considerable interest for the development of any tooth-colored material (Fig 3-51).[12,13] Master ceramists and manufacturers of dental porcelains devote significant time and effort to developing powders that will mimic these two main

3 Conventional Shade Matching

constituents of natural teeth.[14] However, ceramics are used to veneer a metal or ceramic framework in thin layers—a configuration that does not correspond to the arrangement of natural tissues. The anatomy of composite restorations, on the other hand, more closely resembles that of a natural tooth; therefore, the natural tooth can be used as a model for analyzing or developing a composite system.

Specific layering concepts

Four different layering concepts have guided manufacturers in the development of their composite materials.[15] Each concept is based on the specific arrangement of the two or three layers usually needed for large Class 3 and 4 restorations or incisal buildups.

1. *Basic layering concept.* Includes one or two sets of shaded materials (with different opacities but the same chroma range) for the main restoration volume, completed by a limited number of incisal or transparent materials (eg, Prodigy [Kerr, Orange, CA]) (Fig 3-52).
2. *Classic layering concept.* Provides one basic set of shaded materials for dentin replacement (with approximately the same opacity and chroma) and two layers of enamel replacement materials, including shaded enamel and incisal materials (eg, Herculite [Kerr]) (Fig 3-53).
3. *Modern layering concept.* Uses two shaded materials (with different opacity levels) for the replacement of dentin as well as a series of enamel materials (eg, Esthet.x [Dentsply, York, PA]) (Fig 3-54).
4. *Trendy layering concept.* This is the most recent but certainly the most promising concept. It relies on the application of two basic dentin and enamel materials that closely replicate the optical properties of natural tissues and allows for effect materials to be placed between them to create a spatial arrangement that is identical to natural tooth anatomy (eg, Miris [Coltène/Whaledent, Cuyahoga Falls, OH] or Vitalescence [Ultradent, South Jordan, UT]) (Fig 3-55). Shaded dentin materials are available in a single hue (ie, the universal dentin shade, close to Vita A) with a large range of chroma (usually beyond the existing Vita range) and exhibit an opacity close to that of natural dentin. The use of intensive colors or effect materials helps to replicate specific anatomic peculiarities and improve final esthetic outcome. The most useful effect materials are blues (reinforcement of composite natural opalescence), gold-yellows (for a local increase of restoration chroma), and whites (for simulating white spots or hypocalcifications) (Fig 3-56). This approach not only is clinically appropriate but also has excellent esthetic potential.

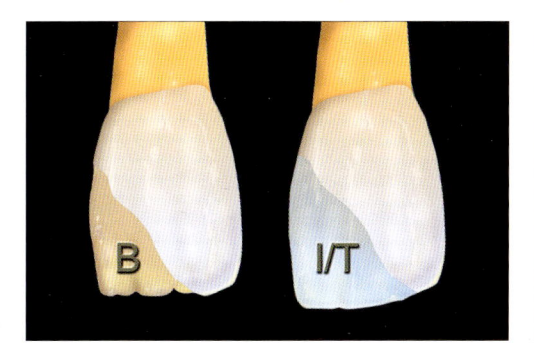

SPECIAL CONSIDERATIONS FOR DIRECT COMPOSITES

Fig 3-52
Basic layering concept. The body material (B) is covered by an incisal or transparent material (I/T).

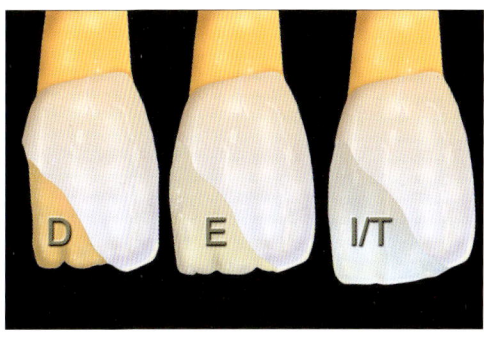

Fig 3-53
Classic layering concept. The bulk of the restoration is made of two colored materials with differing opacities. The first, dentin (D), is more opaque and has a higher chroma; the second is a so-called enamel (E). Finally, the surface is covered by an incisal or transparent material (I/T).

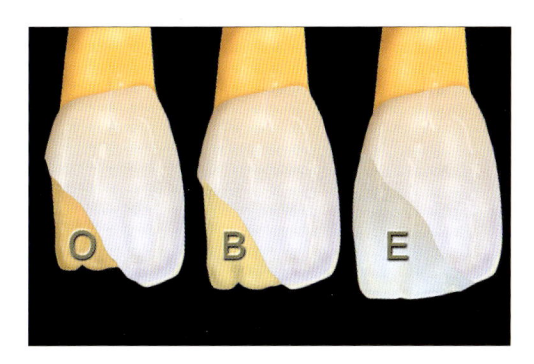

Fig 3-54
Modern layering concept. There are two dentin materials: The first is opaque (O) and is placed in the most interior part of the preparation; the second is less opaque and is used as the body material (B). Enamel materials (E) are used on the surface.

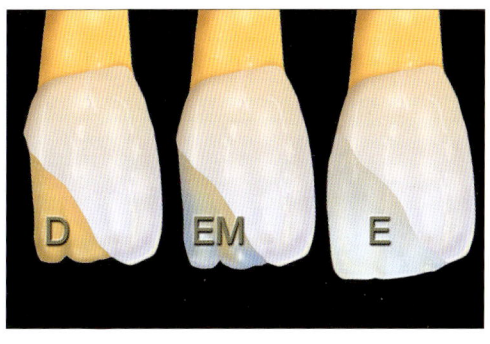

Fig 3-55
Trendy layering concept. The restoration is made from two distinct materials that mimic the position and optical properties of dentin (D) and enamel (E). Effect materials (EM), which are placed between the dentin and enamel materials, complete the system and provide improved esthetics.

Fig 3-56
Miris shade guides for internal characterization (ie, effect materials).

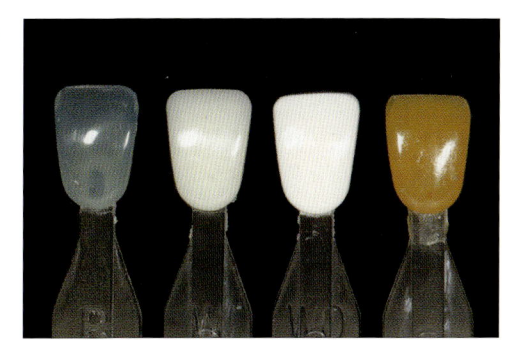

71

3 Conventional Shade Matching

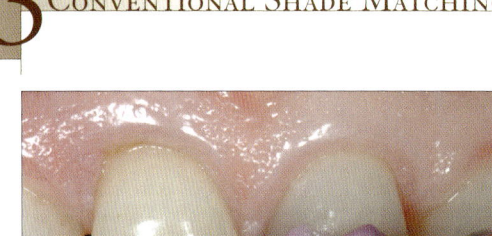

Fig 3-57
Teeth are cleaned with a nonfluoridated prophylaxis paste.

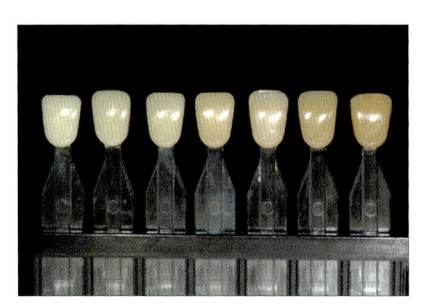

Fig 3-58
Miris shade guide for dentin, following the natural layering concept.

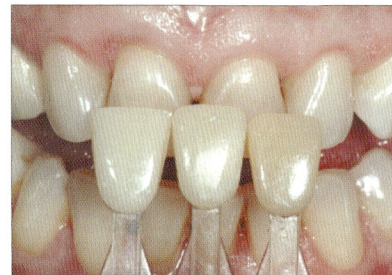

Fig 3-59
Selection of dentinal chroma. A series of dentin tabs are placed close to the tooth in order to determine the most appropriate dentinal chroma.

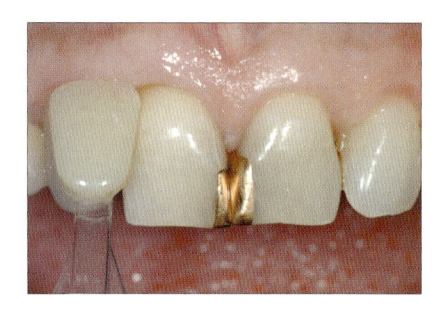

Fig 3-60
The choice of dentinal chroma is confirmed by placing the composite tab close to the cervical area, where there is the least amount of enamel.

Shade selection protocol

According to the natural layering concept, the following four steps should be involved in shade selection for direct composite restorations:

1. Cleaning of the teeth using a prophylaxis paste (Fig 3-57)
2. Selection of dentinal chroma in the cervical area (where enamel is thinnest) using samples of the composite material (Figs 3-58 to 3-60)
3. Selection of enamel tint and translucency by simple visual observation (Fig 3-61)
4. Combination of both samples to demonstrate the final restorative effect and confirm an esthetic match (Figs 3-62 to 3-64)

Figures 3-65 to 3-71 present the shade selection for a case in which the trendy layering concept was used in the direct composite buildup of a peg-shaped lateral incisor.

Special Considerations for Direct Composites

Fig 3-61
Miris shade guide for enamel. The enamel shade tab is selected by visual observation. No attempt is made to select enamel by comparing the composite sample with the tooth.

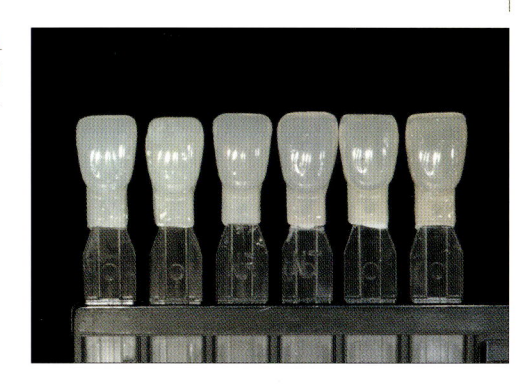

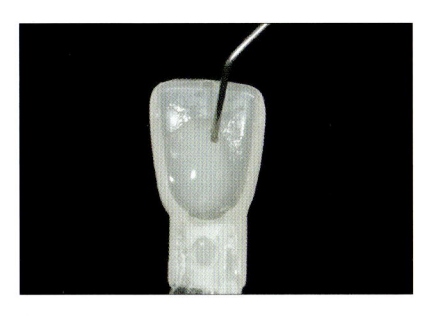

Fig 3-62
A thin layer of glycerine gel is placed in the selected enamel shade tab before the dentin tab is inserted.

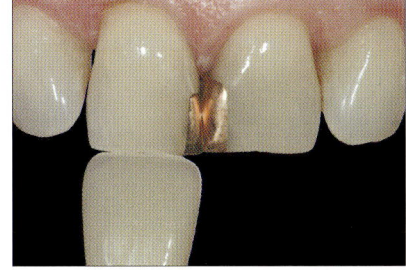

Fig 3-63
The combined enamel and dentin shade tabs are compared to the teeth to determine whether there is an accurate shade match.

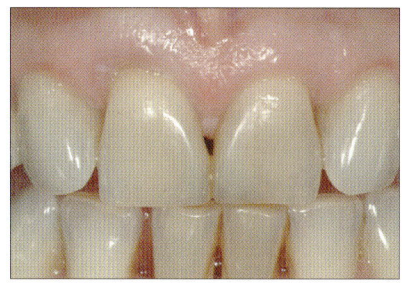

Fig 3-64
Result after 2 years.

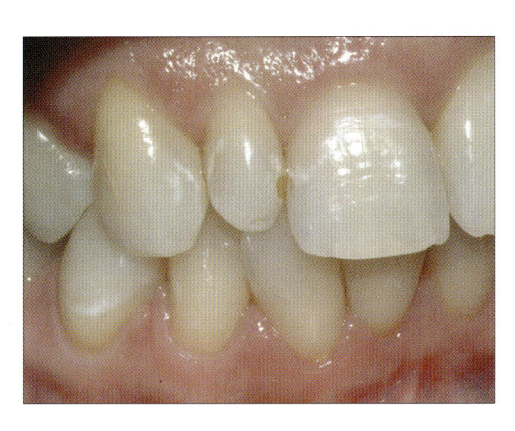

Fig 3-65
Preoperative view of a peg-shaped maxillary right lateral incisor with a discolored mesial restoration.

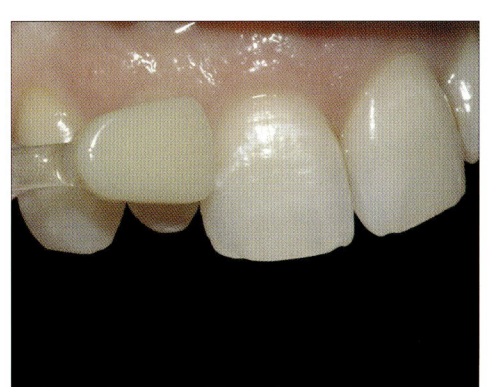

Fig 3-66
Dentin shade selection.

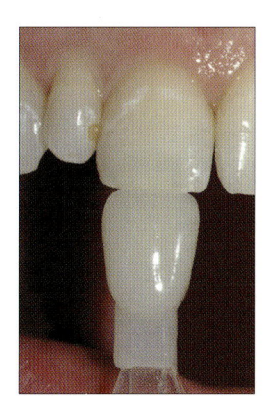

Fig 3-67
The enamel shade with the dentin tab inserted (using glycerin gel) is compared to the tooth to be matched.

73

3 Conventional Shade Matching

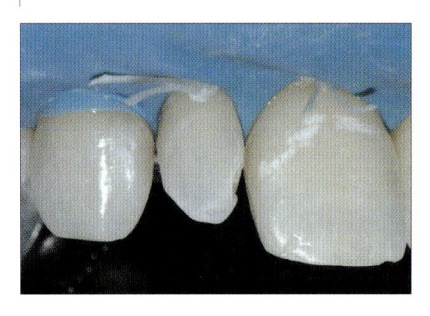

Fig 3-68
Lateral incisor following decay excavation.

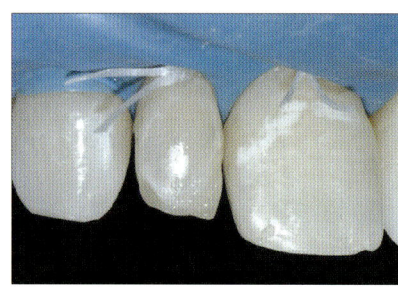

Fig 3-69
Buildup of palatal enamel wall.

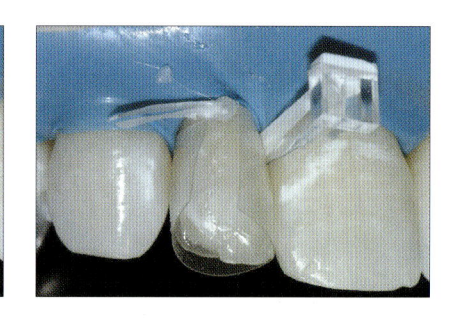

Fig 3-70
Buildup of dentin and labial enamel following the natural layering concept (note the use of blue effect materials next to the incisal edge).

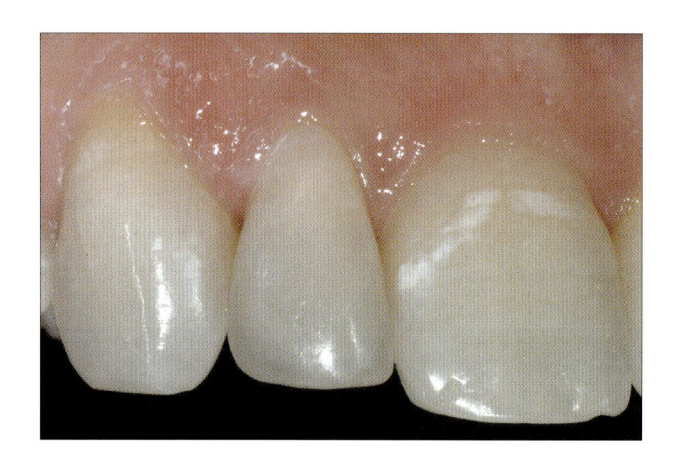

Fig 3-71
Postoperative view.

Conclusions

When tooth shade is selected using conventional means, the knowledge and skill of each practitioner always comes into play. With such a high degree of subjectivity comes significant variability in shade assessment. The development of new restorative materials with improved physical and optical properties also highlights the need for improved methods of shade selection. Both of these factors, as well as clinicians' frustration with wasted chair time due to repeated remakes and the associated loss of productivity,[5] have led to the need for a more objective method of shade matching.

Summary

- Conventional methods are the most common approach to shade matching; however, they involve a high degree of subjectivity, which often leads to unsuccessful shade matches and reduced productivity.
- Traditional shade guides that are currently available use several different methods for quantifying shade.
- For best results with conventional shade matching, the clinician should supply the lab technician with at least eight reference photographs: *(1)* full face; *(2)* full smile; and the teeth to be matched next to the selected *(3)* gingival, *(4)* body, and *(5)* incisal shade tabs, as well as *(6)* an aggregate photograph of all three shade tabs, *(7)* a much brighter shade tab, and *(8)* a much darker shade tab.

Acknowledgments

Photos in Figs 3-14 to 3-16, 3-23 to 3-36, 3-38, 3-43a, 3-43c, and 3-45 to 3-50 courtesy of Irfan Ahmad, BDS, Middlesex, UK.

Text and photos in the section "Special Considerations for Direct Composites" courtesy of Didier Dietschi, DMD, PhD; Stephano Ardu, DMD; and Ivo Krejci, DMD, PhD, Geneva, Switzerland.

References

1. Miller LL. A Scientific Approach to Shade Matching. Chicago: Quintessence, 1988.
2. Avery D. New shade-matching technology: The final piece of the shade communication puzzle. J Dent Technol 2003;20(6):34–35.
3. Miller LL. Shade matching. J Esthet Dent 1993;5(4):143–153.
4. Miller LL. Shade selection. J Esthet Dent 1994;6(2):47–60.
5. Chu SJ. Color. In: Gürel G (ed). The Science and Art of Porcelain Laminate Veneers. Chicago: Quintessence, 2003:158–206.
6. McLaren EA. Provisionalization and the 3-D communication of shade and shape. Contemp Esthet Restorative Pract 2000;May:48–60.
7. Dietschi D. Free-hand composite resin restorations: A key to anterior aesthetics. Pract Periodontics Aesthet Dent 1995;7(7):15–27.
8. Fahl N. Optimizing the esthetics of Class IV restorations with composite resins. J Can Dent Assoc 1997;63(2):108–115.

9. Dietschi D, Dietschi JM. Current developments in composite materials and techniques. Pract Periodontics Aesthet Dent 1996;8:603–614.
10. Dietschi D. Free-hand bonding in the esthetic treatment of anterior teeth: Creating the illusion. J Esthet Dent 1997;9(4):156–164.
11. Dietschi D, Ardu S, Krejci I. Exploring the layering concepts for anterior teeth. In: Roulet JF, Degrange M (eds). Adhesion: The Silent Revolution in Dentistry. Chicago: Quintessence, 2000:235–251.
12. Winter R. Visualizing the natural dentition. J Esthet Dent 1993;5(3):102–117.
13. Chiche G, Pinault A. Esthetics of Anterior Fixed Prosthodontics. Chicago: Quintessence, 1994.
14. Sieber C. Voyage. Chicago: Quintessence, 1994.
15. Dietschi D. Layering concepts in anterior composite restorations. J Adhes Dent 2001;3:71–80.

4 Technology-Based Shade Matching

In this chapter:
- Development of technological shade systems
- Measurement systems
- Types of technological shade systems
- Step-by-step process
- Recommended protocol
- Specifications for currently available technological shade systems

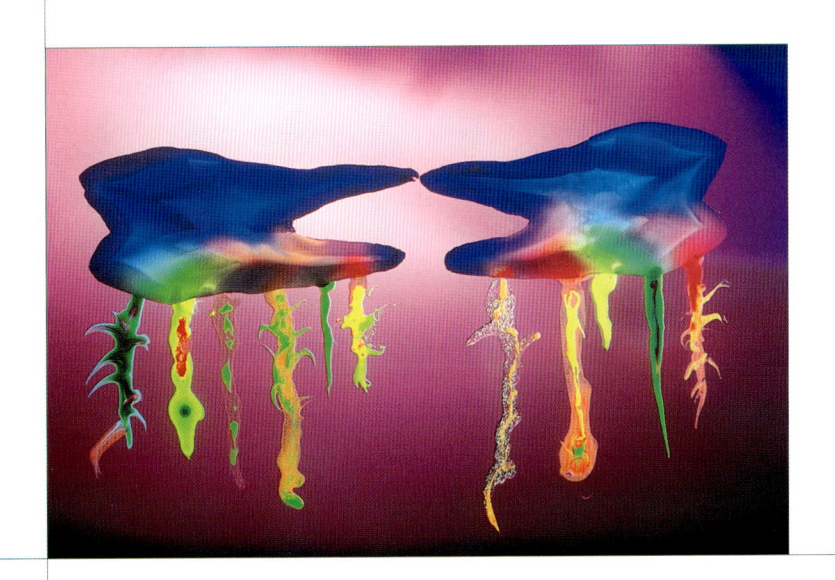

4 Technology-Based Shade Matching

Precise color communication is integral to the development of esthetic harmony and overall restorative success. While traditional shade-taking procedures have enabled some degree of shade information transfer, computerized shade-analysis devices allow for standardized, repeatable shade determinations for increased accuracy by placing technology in the role of "observer" in the light-object-observer triad required for color perception (see chapter 1). Several clinical studies have confirmed that computer-assisted shade analysis is more accurate and more consistent compared with human shade assessment.[1] The need for improvement in the accuracy of shade matching was highlighted by a study that showed that 80% of patients can notice a difference in the shade of their natural teeth compared with their restorations.[2] This widespread lack of accuracy in shade matching should not be accepted as the standard; rather, clinicians should strive to improve the esthetic quality of restorative work.

Advantages of technology-based shade determination:
- No influence of surroundings
- No influence of lighting
- Results are reproducible

Development of Technological Shade Systems

Advancements in technology in the area of computers, the Internet, and communication systems have greatly affected and shaped modern society. Commensurate with these strides are the advancements in contemporary dentistry. During the past half decade, the dental profession has experienced the growth of a new generation of technologies devoted to the analysis, communication, and verification of shade.

Shade determination for direct and indirect restorations has always been a challenge for the esthetic restorative dentist because of the abstract nature of color science. For years, prominent color science experts, such as Bergen, Preston, Miller, and Yamamoto, have attempted to find ways to more objectively quantify color. Bergen experimented with spectrophotometers and computers in an effort to standardize analysis in the profession.[3] Miller used a single-point-source spectrophotometer in his research on correlating the shades of extracted natural teeth to those of available shade guide tabs.[4] Preston identified the quantity and quality of lighting required to analyze shade properly, as well as inconsistencies in the manufacturing of shade guides and tabs.[5] Yamamoto was

Development of Technological Shade Systems

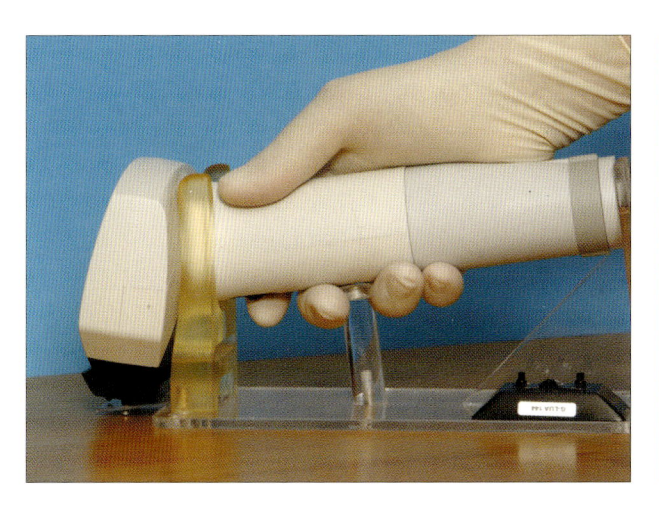

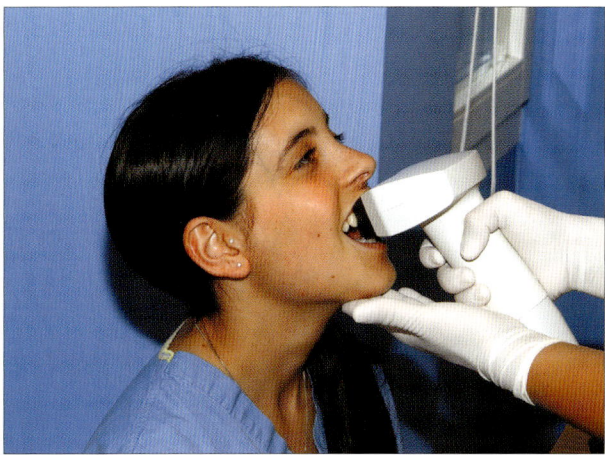

Figs 4-1 and 4-2
The SpectroShade System was the second commercially available system that maps the whole tooth surface.

instrumental in the development of the Shofu ShadeEye Chroma Meter, and subsequently the Shofu NCC (natural color concept) system.[6]

In the late 1990s, a company called Cortex Machina was established in Montreal, Canada, marking the birth of a new industry in dentistry—commercially available technology-based shade guide systems. Cortex Machina, a company devoted to artificial vision technologies and founded by a group of highly trained experts from McGill and Cornell Universities, was approached by a dental technician, Denis Robert, who explained the problems encountered in shade taking and communication between clinician and technician. The shade analysis technology subsequently developed by the company was the first effort toward a complete analysis system that registers shade over the entire tooth surface. Chu and Tarnow[7] reported the clinical use and application of the Cortex Machina prototype, which employed RGB digital camera technology that inferred color properties, in a case study comparing conventional and technology-based shade information in the restoration of a single maxillary central incisor. The authors found that the more accurate data provided by technology-based systems allowed technicians at all levels of skill and experience to produce well-matched restorations. Cortex Machina has subsequently merged with another Canadian company, Cynovad, which specializes in CAD/CAM technologies. The first measurement analysis systems mapping the whole surface of the tooth were the SpectroShade system (a spectrophotometer) from MHT Optic Research in 2001 (Figs 4-1 and 4-2) and the ShadeVision system (a colorimeter) from X-Rite in 2002 (Figs 4-3 and 4-4).

4 Technology-Based Shade Matching

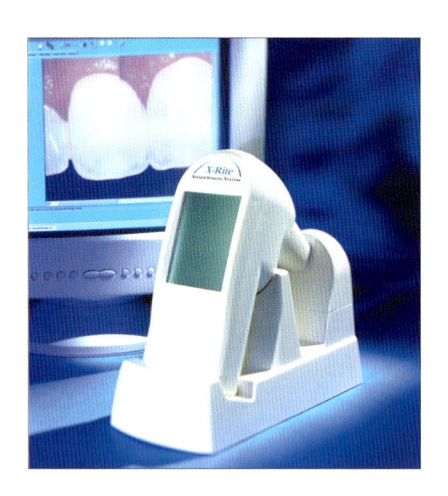

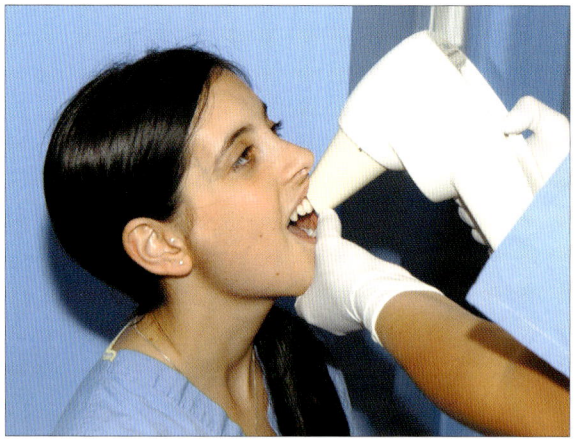

Figs 4-3 and 4-4
ShadeVision stores hue, value, and chroma to efficiently measure tooth shade. Its optical capture device is small, light, and easily maneuverable, allowing image capture in areas beyond the anterior dentition.

Today's digital shade analysis systems seek to mimic the human visual system while eliminating the influence of negative visual illusion effects to deliver exact and reproducible information that will allow the lab technician to produce accurately matched restorations. (See Table 4-1 at the end of the chapter for specifications of the systems currently available.) Additionally, digital shade-taking devices can be used to record the outcome of whitening treatments.

Measurement Systems

Spot measurement (SM) devices measure a small area on the tooth surface, while complete-tooth measurement (CTM) devices measure the entire tooth. For SM devices, the size or diameter of the optical device aperture (generally about 3 mm^2) will determine how much of the tooth surface and subsequent shade is measured (the average central incisor tooth is 80 to 100 mm^2 in area) (Figs 4-5 and 4-6). To create a comprehensive shade map of the entire tooth, the dental professional can obtain several reference measurements with an SM device, although the data may not be entirely accurate because of the nonhomogenous shade structure of the human tooth. Therefore, SM devices are best suited for showing shade trends or tendencies and as adjunct tools in the shade-matching

MEASUREMENT SYSTEMS

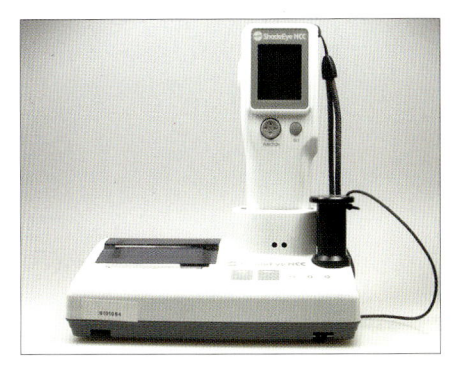

Fig 4-5
The Shofu ShadeEye-NCC system (a spot measurement [SM] device).

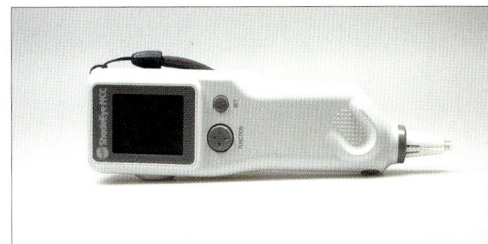

Fig 4-6
On the ShadeEye-NCC, the optical capture device is located on the tip of the instrument, which is about 3 mm² in diameter. To obtain sufficient points of reference for complete shade analysis, a total of nine spot measurements (three each for the gingival, body, and incisal areas) need to be performed. This can be time consuming and increases the potential for tooth dehydration and errors in image capture.

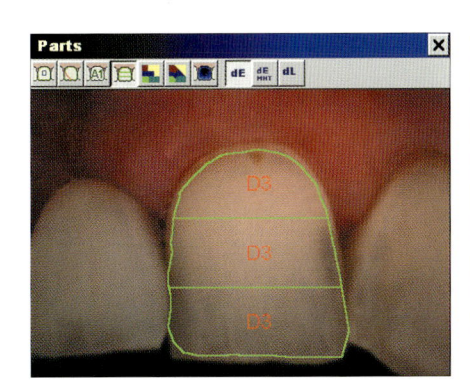

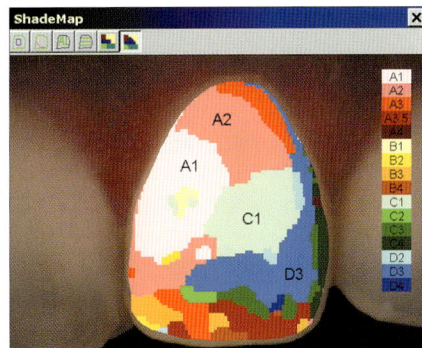

Figs 4-7 and 4-8
Complete-tooth measurement (CTM) devices measure the entire surface of the tooth and provide a detailed color distribution map.

process. Examples of such SM technologies are the Shofu ShadeEye-NCC Chroma Meter system and the Vita Easyshade system.

CTM systems measure the entire tooth surface and provide a topographical color map of the tooth in one image (Figs 4-7 and 4-8). The measurement of the complete surface gives the operator more consistent and reproducible information about the tooth structure[1] (Chu SJ et al, unpublished data, 2004), which then can be transmitted to the lab.

CTM devices offer more convenience and more reliable data when compared with SM devices. In addition, most CTM and SM units are comparable in price, giving CTM devices a better overall cost-benefit ratio.

4 Technology-Based Shade Matching

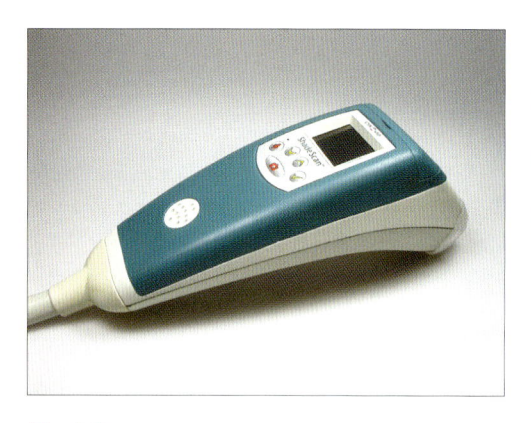

Fig 4-9
The ShadeScan System from Cynovad is an RGB device that functions by inferring the color properties of a tooth.

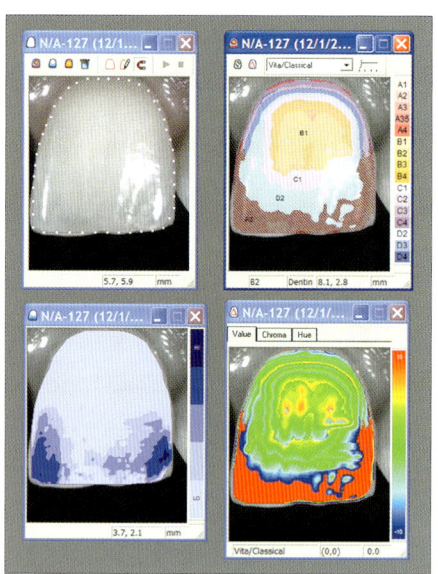

Fig 4-10
A ShadeScan report generated after image capture and data analysis.

Types of Technological Shade Systems

RGB devices

Devices that acquire red, green, and blue image information to create a color image, such as most consumer video or digital still cameras, are commonly referred to as *RGB devices*. Digital cameras and other RGB devices represent the most basic approach to electronic shade taking and still require a certain degree of subjective shade verification by the human eye.[1]

Various approaches have been used to translate this data into useful dental color information.[8] However, the inherent problem with these systems is that they do not control some of the key variables associated with accurate color determination. Typically, color is synthesized from RGB data using various assumptions about the camera and reference materials within the captured image. The information accuracy (reliability) of RGB devices is questionable since they are not measurement instruments; rather, they infer the color properties of the captured image. These systems are useful for providing lab technicians with a referential starting point, but should not be relied upon solely to determine the shade of a tooth. The ShadeScan system from Cynovad is an example of an RGB device (Figs 4-9 and 4-10).

TYPES OF TECHNOLOGICAL SHADE SYSTEMS

Fig 4-11
Digital cameras are useful for taking reference photographs, which are critically important for shade communication. Using lateral flashes helps create more depth and structure in the image.

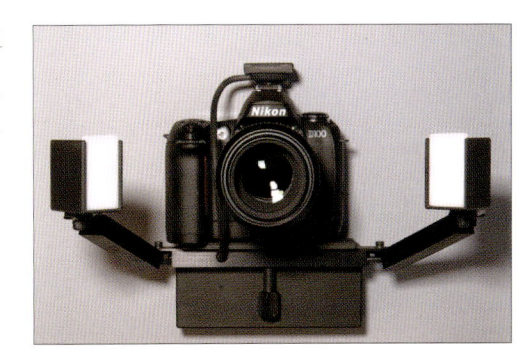

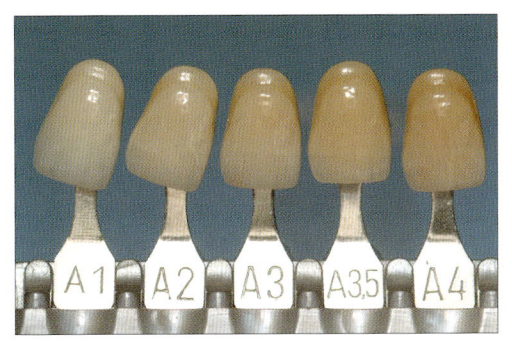

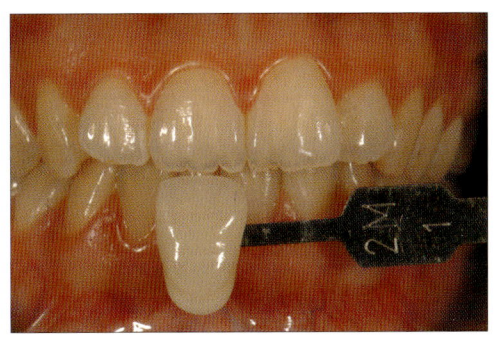

Figs 4-12 and 4-13
Digital images of traditional shade tabs can be used as reference tools to enhance communication between the clinician and the dental technician.

Digital cameras

Although still not used predominately in dentistry, digital photography is gaining popularity at an extraordinary rate throughout the world. At present, the use of digital photography in dentistry has no set nomenclature, procedure codes, standards, or continuity.

Digital photography, like many of the newer electronic technologies in the industry, offers significant benefits to dental practices. The digital camera is extremely efficient and easy to use; however, the practitioner needs a basic understanding of computer technology and photographic methods to maximize its capabilities (Fig 4-11). Training staff members to acquire and manipulate the images can make the process cost effective and beneficial to both the practice and the patient.[9] Digital photography can be an ideal supplement for the clinician and lab technician in quantifying shade; eg, these systems are often used for reference photographs in conjunction with traditional shade tabs to enhance the communication between the clinician and the lab technician (Figs 4-12 and 4-13). Also,

83

4 Technology-Based Shade Matching

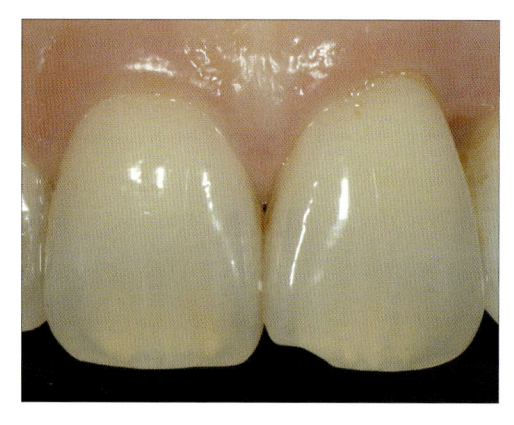

Fig 4-14
Teeth that are high in translucency are generally perceived as darker.

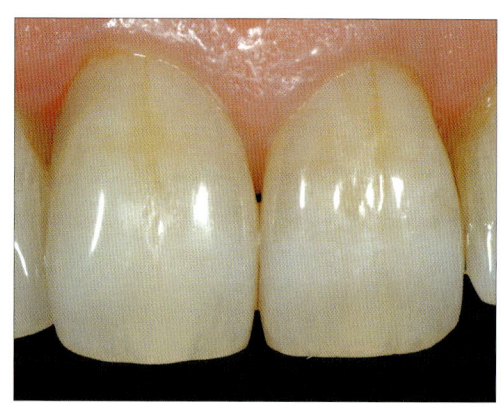

Fig 4-15
Teeth that are high in opacity are generally perceived as whiter.

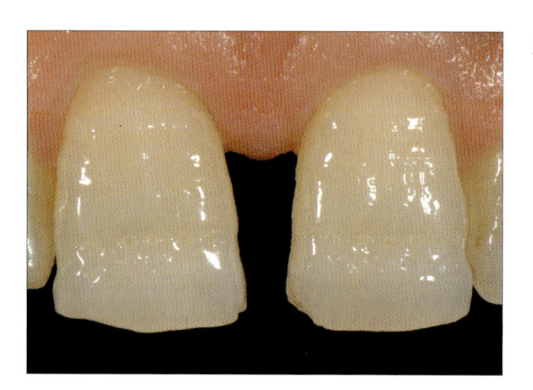

Fig 4-16
The surface texture of teeth can also affect their perceived color.

reference photographs can reveal the translucency and opacity (Figs 4-14 and 4-15) as well as the surface texture of teeth (Fig 4-16), all of which may affect the perceived and recorded shade of the teeth. This information is important for the lab technician, who will be able to incorporate these characteristics into the restoration, resulting in an improved esthetic result. However, the use of a digital camera alone is not effective for shade analysis.

It is important to remember that individual digital cameras, like individual people, interpret color differently, making standardization very difficult to achieve. In addition, factors such as illumination and the angle of the photograph will alter how color is perceived by the camera. Therefore, it is important to use digital photography only as an adjunct to other techniques and to take several reference photographs using consistent illumination to provide sufficient information for shade analysis.

TYPES OF TECHNOLOGICAL SHADE SYSTEMS

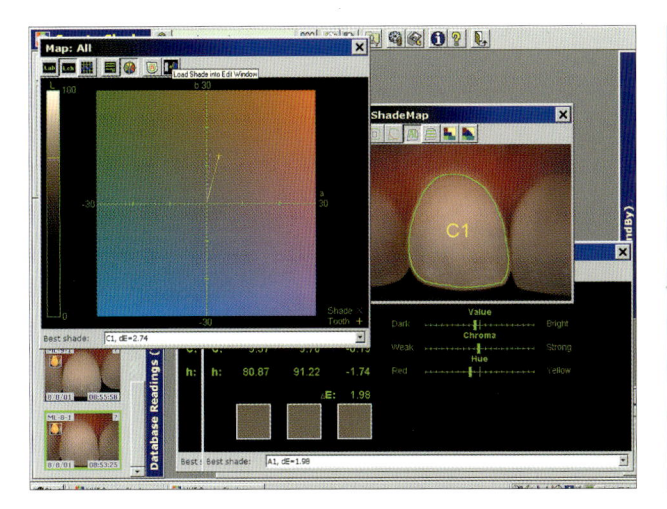

Fig 4-17
Data obtained from spectrophotometers are often difficult to translate into everyday dentistry. However, scientific parameters and data output by such devices are highly useful in the research arena.

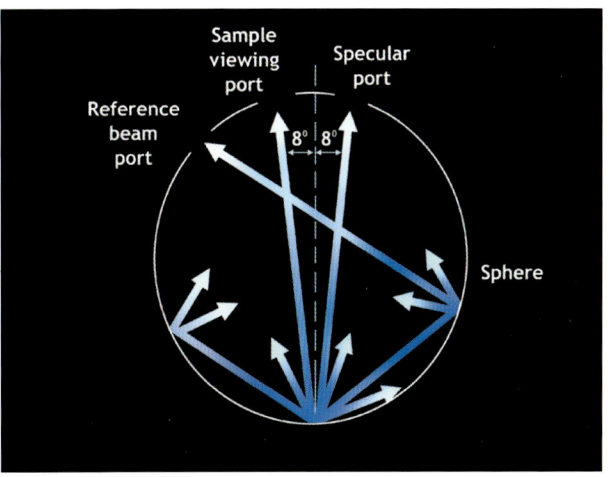

Fig 4-18
Effective laboratory research-based spectrophotometers use spherical optics technology. This 360-degree light exposure is not achievable for dental purposes.

Spectrophotometers

A spectrophotometer measures and records the amount of visible radiant energy reflected or transmitted by an object one wavelength at a time for each value, chroma, and hue present in the entire visible spectrum.[1,2,10–13] The extensive data obtained from spectrophotometers must be manipulated, and a data-reduction strategy employed, to translate the data into a useful format, eg, a spectral curve (Fig 4-17).[14]

Widespread use of spectrophotometers in dental research and clinical settings has been hindered by the fact that the equipment is expensive and complex, and that, until recently, it was difficult to measure the color of teeth in vivo with these machines. The best research spectrophotometer uses what is called *spherical optics*, in which the object is placed inside the spectrophotometer and exposed to light from many different angles and directions (Fig 4-18). This gives the most accurate and precise spectral analysis of the reflectance properties of the object. However, spectrophotometers for dental use cannot achieve this same 360-degree light exposure since the tooth cannot be placed inside the device. Instead, light is directed at the surface of the tooth.

There are two basic optical light settings used in reflectance spectrophotometer instruments: illumination at 0 degrees and observation at 45 degrees

85

4 Technology-Based Shade Matching

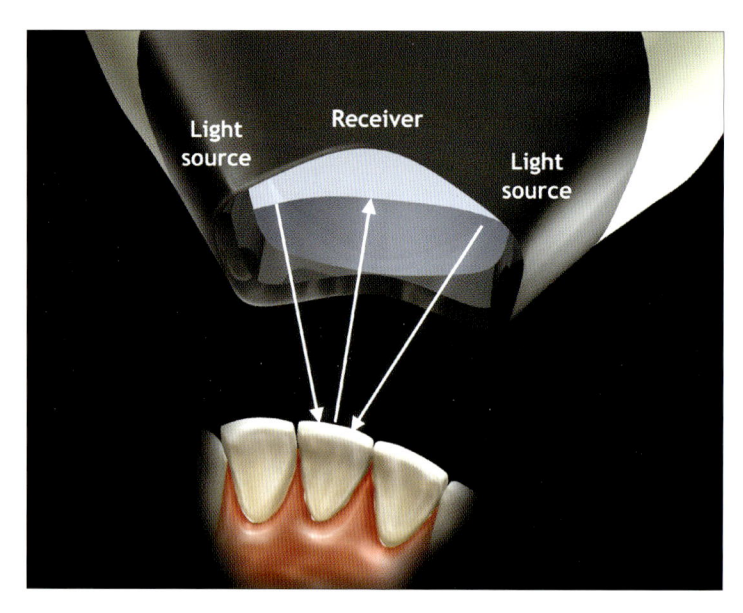

Fig 4-19
The 45/0 option (illumination at 45 degrees and observation at 0 degrees) is best suited for clinical use of spectrophotometers.

(0/45) or illumination at 45 degrees and observation at 0 degrees (45/0). Because of the limited access afforded by the oral cavity, only the 45/0 option is suitable for clinical use (Fig 4-19).

An example of a spectrophotometer developed for clinical use is the SpectroShade from MHT. The SpectroShade system uses dual digital cameras linked through optic fibers to the spectrophotometer to measure the color of the tooth. There is a multimodal dual-light mechanism that illuminates the tooth and allows readings of its translucency and reflectivity.[15] The SpectroShade has the capability to display shade results in advanced color graphics.

Colorimeters

Much of the dental research on the color of natural teeth and porcelains, in vivo and in vitro, has been conducted using colorimeters.[16–20] These instruments are engineered to directly measure color as perceived by the human eye. A colorimeter filters light in three or four areas of the visible spectrum to determine the color of an object. Colorimeters are difficult to design and, if made improperly, will result in reduced accuracy compared with a spectrophotometer. However, well-designed colorimeters such as X-Rite's ShadeVision system can provide greater data efficiency because they only store the three data points of hue, value, and chroma instead of the 16 or more data points of reflectance recorded by a spectrophotometer.[1] In addition, a colorimeter can deliver color information accuracy similar to spectrophotometers while reducing the data load time by avoiding the unnecessary color mapping associated with spectrophotometers. The ShadeVision system provides simple, consistently reliable shade measurement information for precise, quantifiable communications between the dental office and laboratory, significantly improving the assurance of an accurate shade match when compared with traditional techniques.

As discussed previously, a hydrated tooth surface has a significant impact on the perceived shade, particularly in terms of value. The smoother (more reflective) the surface is, the brighter the surface will appear. To overcome this problem, some systems use filters to eliminate the surface gloss. Shade-matching systems that do not use such filters often record shades at a value that is too high, which can be very problematic.

Step-by-Step Process

Analysis

Most technology-based shade systems use the ΔE from the *Commission Internationale de l'Éclairage* (CIE) $L^*a^*b^*$ color system to determine the color difference between a tooth to be matched and a chosen shade. The ΔE is the shortest distance in the CIE $L^*a^*b^*$ color space between the colors being compared, as determined by the following equation:

$$\Delta E = (\Delta L^{*2} + \Delta a^{*2} + \Delta b^{*2})^{1/2}$$

where L^* represents *lightness* (from white to black; similar to value), a^* corresponds to the red-green axis (positive value indicates red; negative indicates green), and b^* corresponds to the yellow-blue axis (a positive value indicates yellow; negative indicates blue). The ΔL, Δa, and Δb, as well as the total ΔE, are shown graphically with the ShadeVision and ShadeEye systems and in a numeric form with the SpectroShade system. Additionally, the SpectroShade system allows the dental professional to change the selected shade according to different ΔEs, which improves accuracy in the initial shade selection (Fig 4-20).

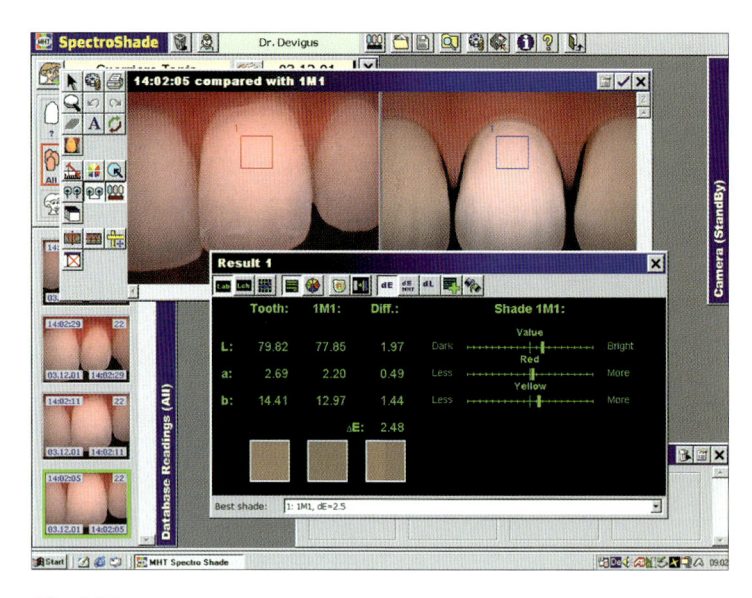

4 Technology-Based Shade Matching

Fig 4-20
The ΔE value obtained with the SpectroShade system provides quantification of the shade difference between a selected shade and the shade to be matched. The smallest ΔE value is ideal since it implies the closest match. The ShadeVision system is also capable of providing such ΔE data through a special software program called *ShadeMatch*.

With digital shade analysis, the goal is to achieve the smallest ΔE value possible, indicating the most accurate shade match, for the gingival, body, and incisal sections of the tooth. It is important to note that ΔE values are nondirectional, ie, they do not indicate whether one shade is darker or lighter than another. The ΔL (value) is the most significant parameter because the human eye can detect changes in value more readily than it can perceive changes in hue. A ΔL of less than 2.0 and a total ΔE of less than 4.0 have been shown to represent clinically acceptable color matching.[1]

Digital shade analysis is much less time consuming and subjective than the conventional approach. The shade is taken electronically, with either a colorimeter or spectrophotometer, and a color map is created automatically, verified visually, and then sent to the lab technician.

Shade analysis also involves the selection of the restorative material to be used. As discussed in chapters 2 and 3, the intrinsic properties of different materials greatly affect the perceived shade of the restoration.

Communication

A high level of communication between the clinician and the lab technician is the basis for predictable results and a successful clinical case. There are two major components to clinician-laboratory communication:

- Administrative communication, eg, payment arrangement, remake policies, delivery schedules, and fees
- Technical communication, eg, study models, diagnostic waxups, occlusal records, shade tabs, computerized shade mapping, and photographs

This text focuses on technical communication, although good administrative communication is also important to a good working relationship with a laboratory.

With technology-based systems, communication is significantly improved and streamlined primarily as a result of the standardized shade-analysis reports, which allow all communication to be done electronically. With the ShadeVision and SpectroShade systems, for example, the images are conveniently captured and the data is uploaded to the clinician's personal computer for processing. This information is easily sent by e-mail or fax to the laboratory, which then has objective data to fabricate and verify the restoration's esthetics.

Even though technology-based systems capture a significant amount of detail and shade information, reference photographs also should be sent with the color data so the lab technician has sufficient information to fabricate the restoration accurately. Technology alone cannot provide enough information to ensure an accurate shade match.

Interpretation

The lab technician analyzes the color map and interprets the reference photographs before fabricating the restoration. Interpretation of technology-based reports is still subjective, and depending upon the knowledge and skill of the lab technician, the reading can be varied. Additionally, the technician must take into account several factors that can modify the perceived color of the restoration, eg, surface texture, anatomic form, surface gloss, and fluorescence.

4 Technology-Based Shade Matching

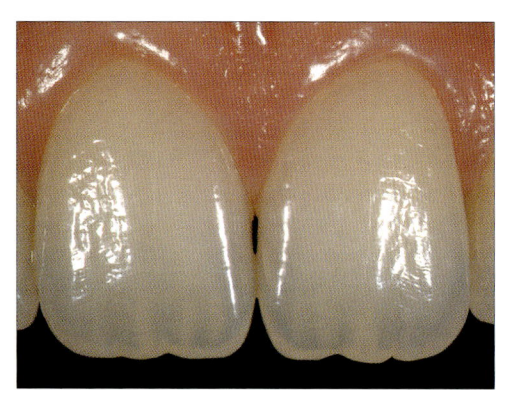

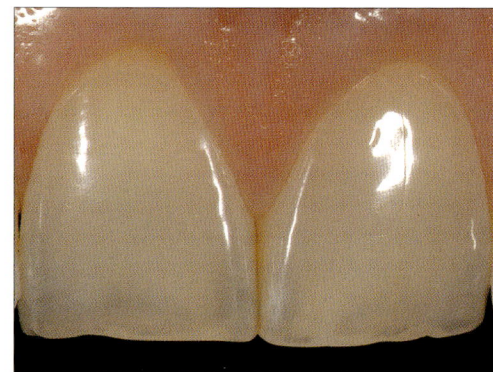

Figs 4-21 and 4-22
When attempting to create a natural-looking restoration, it is important to note that tooth structure varies and changes with age. Figure 4-21 presents the square-shaped morphology characteristic of adolescents' teeth, while Fig 4-22 shows the more tapered and triangular shape of an older patient's teeth.

Fabrication

When fabricating the restoration, the technician must consider the intrinsic properties of the selected restorative material not only to match the shade, but also to achieve the appropriate translucency and opacity. Each tooth presents different levels of translucency, which must be simulated in the restorative material. Extrapolated or inferred translucency maps can be interpreted to determine the ideal amount of translucency and opacity. It is also important to fabricate restorations with a shape and color that appropriately reflect the patient's age. In the oral environment, age-related extrinsic factors, such as changes in the supporting periodontal tissues and wear facets, affect the overall appearance of a tooth.

In adolescents, the morphology of the visible tooth is commonly square (Fig 4-21). With age, dentin becomes more exposed, and there is wear on the incisal edges, causing the tooth to have a more tapered and triangular shape (Fig 4-22). In addition, in adolescence, the surface characteristics are accentuated, with the surface appearing rough. As teeth age, their surface texture becomes more shiny and smooth because of continuous abrasion and attrition.

Aging also affects the color of teeth in the following ways:

- The dentin becomes more visible through the thinner enamel (Fig 4-23).
- Increased calcification results in higher opacity (Fig 4-24).
- The dentin becomes more opaque and darker with age (Fig 4-25).
- The high-value, whitish color of the young patient's teeth changes to a low-value orange, then to a low-value, brownish color with age (Fig 4-26).

Step-by-Step Process

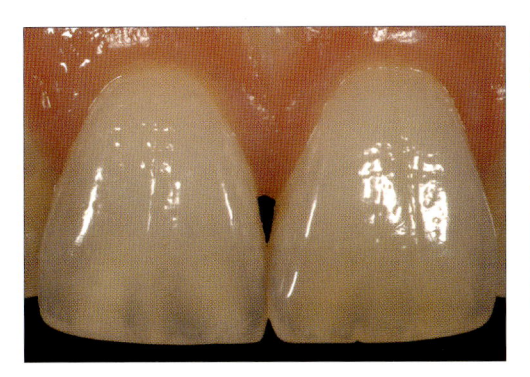

Fig 4-23
In older teeth, dentinal structures are more prominent because of an increased translucency of the enamel, which is caused by abrasion.

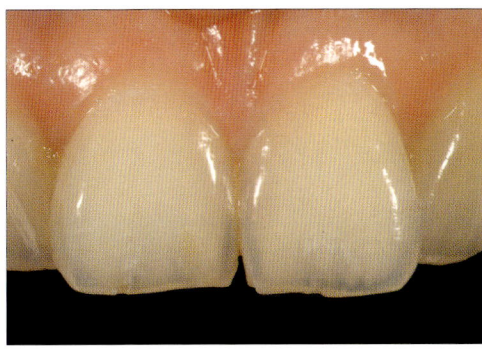

Fig 4-24
Calcification of the teeth leads to higher opacity with age.

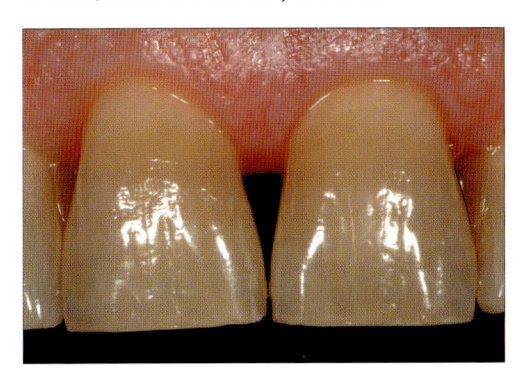

Fig 4-25
Diffusion of light through dentin decreases with age, creating a more opaque appearance and an increasingly saturated hue.

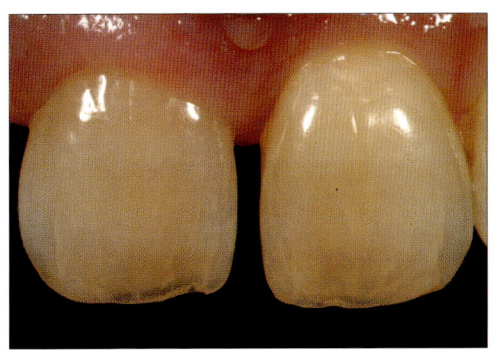

Fig 4-26
Teeth change to a low-value orange, then to a low-value brownish color with age.

Verification

Verifying the shade of the restoration is significantly improved with advanced technology. The ShadeVision system, for example, has a virtual try-in feature, and the SpectroShade system has a restoration verification mode that allows the lab technician to verify the esthetics of the restoration electronically before sending it back to the clinician. This ensures the shade accuracy of the restoration prior to the visit and reduces the number of remakes and wasted patient appointments. Spot measurement devices help the lab technician to verify the shade of a layered ceramic, but only in specific areas, not over the entire surface.

4 Technology-Based Shade Matching

Recommended Protocol (Figs 4-27 to 4-38)

The following recommended protocol is based on the use of ShadeVision technology. Refer to Table 4-1 at the end of the chapter and the clinical cases in the Appendix for more details on other digital shade systems.

In the operatory:

1. Remove the instrument from the docking station.
2. On the instrument's display screen, select the tooth to be measured (Fig 4-27).
3. Use your thumb and forefinger as a fulcrum to aid in aligning the tip against the tooth surface (Figs 4-28 and 4-29).
4. Use direct vision to verify that the tip of the instrument is in the correct position on the tooth surface to be measured. For the most accurate shade reading, the ShadeVision tip must:
   - Rest against the tooth and gingival area, touching the tooth
   - Be flush and square with the tooth surface
   - Be parallel to the long axis of the tooth
5. Press *Target* on the touch screen.
6. Use the line-of-sight viewing window to adjust positioning while the bar graph counts down from 100% to 0%. After it reaches 0%, hold the unit steady until you hear a beep.
7. Review image to confirm that:
   - It is centered on the screen.
   - It is not blurred.
   - There are no artifacts from the tongue, lips, opposing teeth, or operator's fingers.
8. Press *Accept* to proceed or *Cancel* to retake the image.
9. Send the work order to the laboratory via e-mail, on disk, or as a printed copy by fax or regular mail. If the work order arrives by e-mail, the lab technician can simply double-click to download the information to the ShadeVision database (Figs 4-30 to 4-34).

RECOMMENDED PROTOCOL

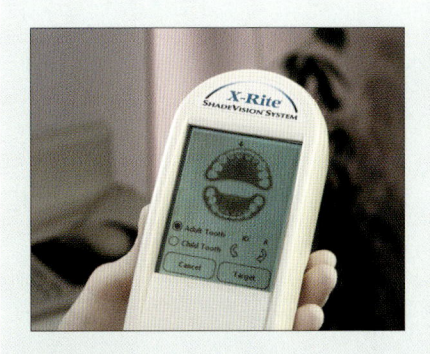

Fig 4-27
Display screen of the ShadeVision instrument on which the tooth to be measured is selected by touch.

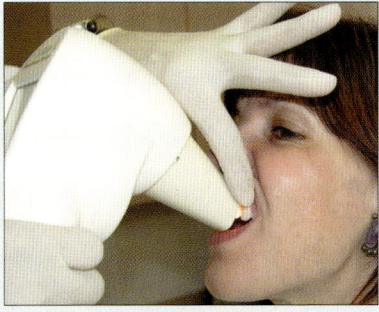

Fig 4-28
The instrument is placed against the tooth surface, using the thumb and forefinger as a fulcrum.

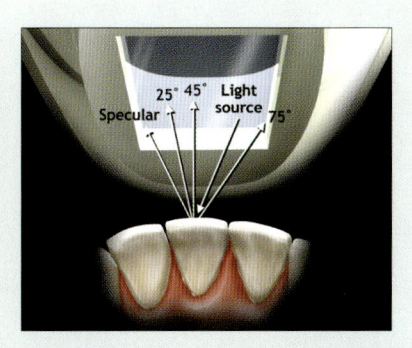

Fig 4-29
The tip of the instrument will read the properties of the tooth through various angles of reflected light.

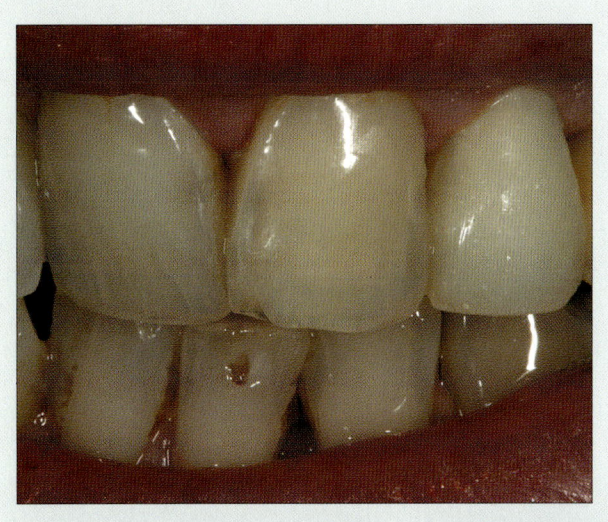

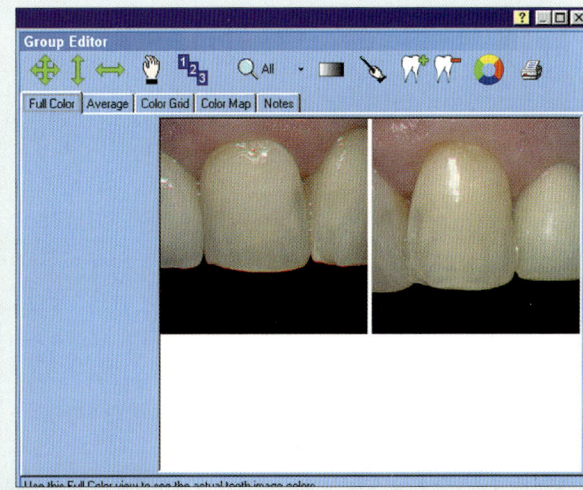

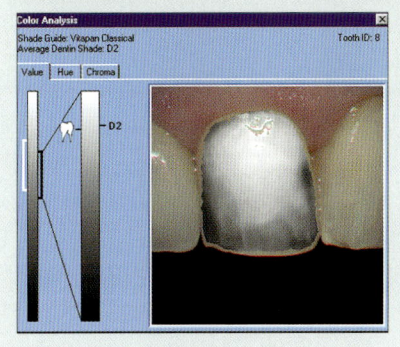

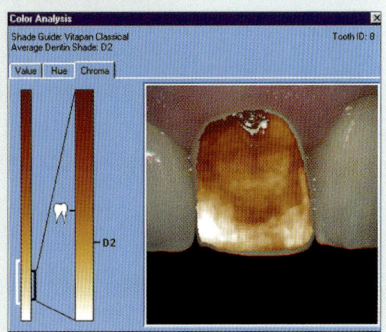

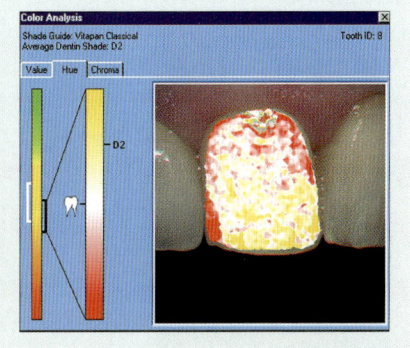

Figs 4-30 to 4-34
With ShadeVision, digital color information can be communicated easily and accurately from the clinician to the lab technician via e-mail.

93

4 Technology-Based Shade Matching

In the laboratory:

10. The lab technician interprets the shade information and fabricates the restoration (Fig 4-35).

Note that the ShadeVision system has an internal software analysis program that automatically defaults to lighter shade data. This affords the clinician and technician the option to increase the chroma and lower the value of the restoration if it is too light. (This is easier than lightening a restoration that is too dark.)

11. The technician places the restoration in the ShadeVision restoration holder, which was designed specifically to assist lab technicians in verifying the accuracy of the restoration's shade, and follows the methods in steps 1 to 8 to check the shade (Fig 4-36).
12. The technician reviews and edits all measured teeth using the ShadeVision software tools, then clicks on the green check to proceed when tooth definition is acceptable.
13. The Creation Restoration Wizard will upload the original images from the clinician, along with the lab technician's restoration image. This virtual try-in feature allows the lab technician to visually check the restoration

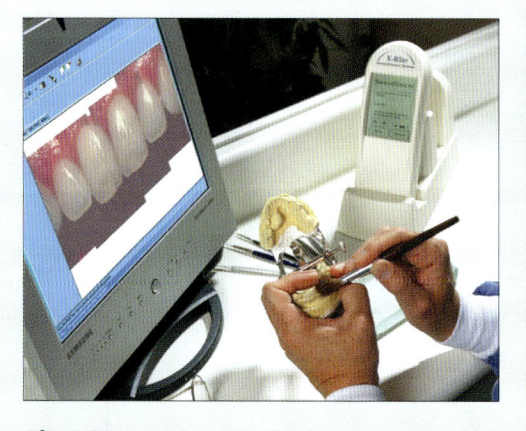

Fig 4-35
The lab technician uses the digital shade data to fabricate the restoration.

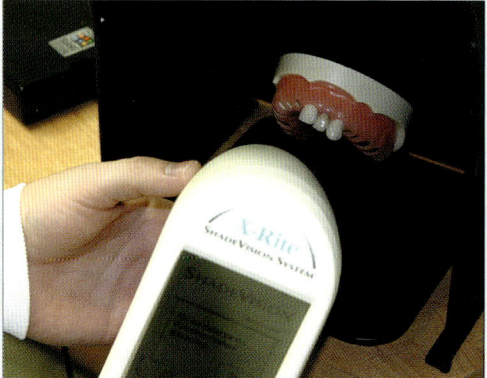

Fig 4-36
The restoration is placed in the restoration holder and scanned in the laboratory.

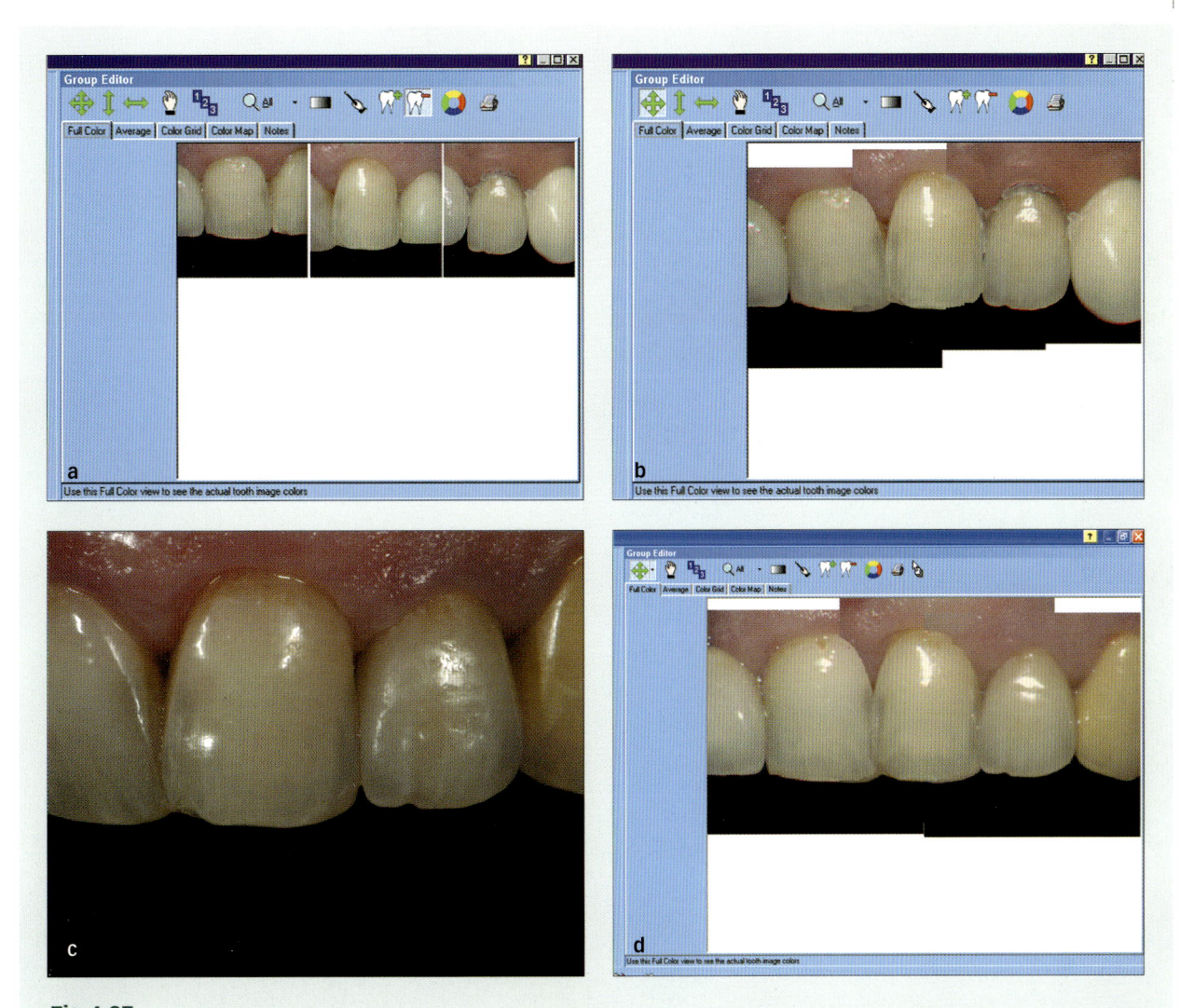

RECOMMENDED PROTOCOL

Fig 4-37
The virtual try-in. This allows the lab technician to verify that the shade matches the tooth before it is sent back to the clinician. This saves time and frustration and increases productivity chairside, thereby making dentistry less stressful and more enjoyable. *(a)* Laboratory virtual try-in before images are combined. *(b)* Laboratory virtual try-in with images combined. *(c)* Clinical photo of restoration in place showing a good visual shade match. *(d)* Virtual try-in mocked up after restoration has been placed. Note how similar this is to the laboratory virtual try-in shown in *(b)*, demonstrating the accuracy of this feature.

against the original images (Fig 4-37). If the match is acceptable on the monitor, it will be acceptable in the mouth. However, achieving a perfect shade match using technology alone is difficult (Fig 4-38).

14. The lab technician confirms the work order information and adds notes to send to the clinician if necessary.

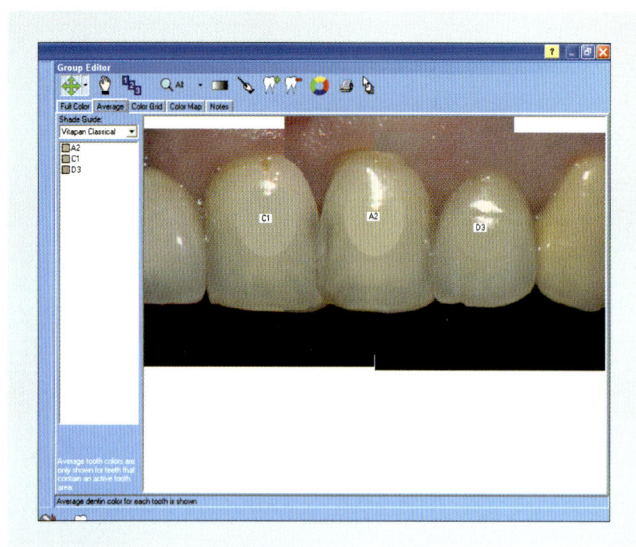

4 Technology-Based Shade Matching

Fig 4-38
Final analysis with the ShadeVision system shows that although the match is clinically acceptable, the restoration does not perfectly match the dentition. The results would have been improved if both conventional and technology-based techniques had been used (see chapter 5).

Conclusions

Technology-based systems provide restorative dentists with a distinct advantage in creating highly esthetic, natural-looking restorations. The reports are less subjective, the capture of an image takes less time, and, with most systems, the shade of a restoration can be verified before it is sent back to the clinician. (See Table 4-1 for a detailed breakdown of the systems currently available.) The current predominant disadvantage of these systems is cost, which might detract from their widespread appeal. Additionally, further clinical studies are necessary to document the effectiveness of digital shade taking. However, the advantages provided by these systems, ie, an unbiased reading of shade and elimination of operatory distractions and the frailties associated with the human visual system, make the investment worthwhile, and, as discussed in the following chapter, quality control can be maintained by pairing technological and conventional shade-matching techniques.

In addition, in the future, technology-based shade-matching systems may be used to standardize the fabrication of ceramic and composite materials, thereby solving some of the current problems caused by inconsistencies in the materials (see chapter 2). The possible applications for these systems will most likely continue to expand; however, it is important to remember that human interpretive skills will never be fully replaced. Only the clinician can achieve a true understanding of the patient's desires through dialogue, and this process will always play an important role in successful treatment.

Summary

- Analysis and communication of shade are enhanced with technology-based systems.
- The three predominant categories of shade-taking technology are RGB devices, spectrophotometers, and colorimeters.
- Digital shade analysis creates a more objective standard for assessing shade, while eliminating the distractions in the operatory.

4 Technology-Based Shade Matching

TABLE 4-1 SPECIFICATIONS FOR CURRENTLY AVAILABLE TECHNOLOGICAL SHADE SYSTEMS*

Product	Company	Measurement	Principle	Portable	PC image	PC software	Virtual try-in
ShadeVision	X-Rite (Grandville, MI)	Complete tooth	Colorimeter	Yes	Yes	Yes	Yes
ShadeScan	Cynovad (Montreal, Canada)	Complete tooth	RGB Digital camera	No	Yes	Yes	No
SpectroShade	MHT Optic Research (Niederhasli, Switzerland)	Complete tooth	Spectro-photometer	No	Yes	Yes	No
ikam	DCM (Leeds, UK)	Complete tooth	RGB Digital camera	No	Yes	Yes	No
ShadeEye-NCC	Shofu (San Marcos, CA)	Spot	Colorimeter	Yes	No	Yes	No
Digital Shade Guide	Rieth (Schorndorf, Germany)	Spot	Colorimeter	No	No	Yes	No
Easyshade	Vita (Bad Sackingen, Germany)	Spot	Spectro-photometer	No	No	Optional	No

*This overview is not intended as a buyer's guide. Its purpose is to show the range of systems currently available on the market. The clinician and lab technician should evaluate each system according to their specific needs prior to making a purchasing decision.

Summary

E-mail capability	Advantages	Disadvantages
Yes	Cordless Good technical phone support Good image quality Automatically defaults to lighter shade to facilitate shade-matching correction Good hue, chroma, and value contrast maps Images can be added from other files Access is not limited to the anterior teeth Disposable image capture tips Restoration shade verification Virtual try-in software program	Only 8 images can be captured before downloading is required LCD screen of optical device is black and white and sometimes hard to read Image capture (especially of mandibular teeth) can be difficult Difficult to image capture severely misaligned teeth
Yes	Good software Enhanced image option Organized printed report Resoration shade verification	Plastic lens protector is easily scratched, can distort images, fogs up, must be sterilized (not disposable) Difficult to get technical support Difficult to image capture severely misaligned teeth
Yes	High-accuracy reference system Measures difference between closest shade tab and actual shade (ΔE) Nearly unlimited number of image captures Can assess bleaching changes very accurately (vertical split-image software) Restoration shade verification	Expensive Large, bulky unit Large optical head can cause patient discomfort Mildly susceptible to fogging Produces matte images only Difficult to image capture severly misaligned teeth
Yes	Works with digital camera Good image quality	Difficult to position patient Bulky device
No	No PC required Direct printout Easy handling Three modes: tooth, porcelain, whitening Comfortable for patient	No overall information Incisal measurement poor System works best with Shofu ceramics
No	Small device Good price	Design is not ergonomic PC-dependent No sterilization
No	Easy handling Comfortable for patient Access to molar region Tooth and ceramic mode	Works only with Vita shades

References

1. Paul S, Peter A, Pietrobon N, Hammerle CH. Visual and spectrophotometric shade analysis of human teeth. J Dent Res 2002;81:578–592.
2. Ishikawa-Nagai S, Sato R, Furukawa K, Ishibashi K. Using a computer color-matching system in color reproduction of porcelain restorations. Part 1: Application of CCM to the opaque layer. Int J Prosthodont 1992;5:495–502.
3. Bergen SF. Color in aesthetics. N Y State Dent J 1985;51:470–471.
4. Miller LL. A scientific approach to shade matching. In: Preston JD (ed). Perspectives in Dental Ceramics: Proceedings of the Fourth International Symposium on Ceramics. Chicago: Quintessence, 1988:193–208.
5. Preston JD. Current status of shade selection and color matching. Quintessence Int 1985;16:47–58.
6. Yamamoto M. Development of the vintage halo computer color search system. Quintessence Dent Technol 1998;21:9–26.
7. Chu SJ, Tarnow DP. Digital shade analysis and verification: A case report and discussion. Pract Periodontics Aesthet Dent 2001;13:129–136.
8. Morris AC, Mabrito CA, Roberts MR [inventors]. Automated tooth shade analysis and matching system. US patent 6,190,170 B1. 20 February 2001.
9. American Dental Association. Proposed American Dental Association Guide to Digital Dental Photography and Imaging [Technical Report No. 1029]. Chicago: American Dental Association, 2003.
10. Trushkowsky RD. How a spectrophotometer can help you achieve esthetic shade matching. Compend Contin Educ Dent 2003;24:60–66.
11. Ishikawa-Nagai S, Sawafuji F, Tsuchitoi H, Sato RR, Ishibashi K. Using a computer color-matching system in color reproduction of porcelain restorations. Part 2: Color reproduction of stratiform-layered porcelain samples. Int J Prosthodont 1993;6:522–527.
12. Ishikawa-Nagai S, Sato RR, Shiraishi A, Ishibashi K. Using a computer color-matching system in color reproduction of porcelain restorations. Part 3: A newly developed spectrophotometer designed for clinical application. Int J Prosthodont 1994;7:50–55.
13. Horn DJ, Bulan-Brady J, Hicks ML. Sphere spectrophotometer versus human evaluation of tooth shade. J Endod 1998;24:786–790.
14. Freedman G. Communicating color. Dent Today 2001;20:76–80.
15. Hunter RS, Harold RW. The Measurement of Appearance, ed 2. New York: John Wiley & Sons, 1987:290–302.
16. Okubo SR, Kananwati A, Richards MW, Childress S. Evaluation of visual and instrument shade matching. J Prosthet Dent 1998;80:642–648.
17. Tung FF, Goldstein GR, Jang S, Hittelman E. The repeatability of an intraoral dental colorimeter. J Prosthet Dent 2002;88:585–590.
18. Yap AU, Sim CP, Loh WL, Teo JH. Human-eye versus computerized color matching. Oper Dent 1999;24:358–363.
19. Swift EJ Jr, Hammel SA, Lund PS. Colorimetric evaluation of Vita shade composites. Int J Prosthodont 1994;7:356–361.
20. Dancy WK, Yaman P, Dennison JB, O'Brien WJ, Razzoog ME. Color measurements as quality criteria for clinical shade matching of porcelain crowns. J Esthet Restor Dent 2003;15:114–121.

5 Recommended Shade-Matching Protocol

In this chapter:
- Seven steps to a successful shade match

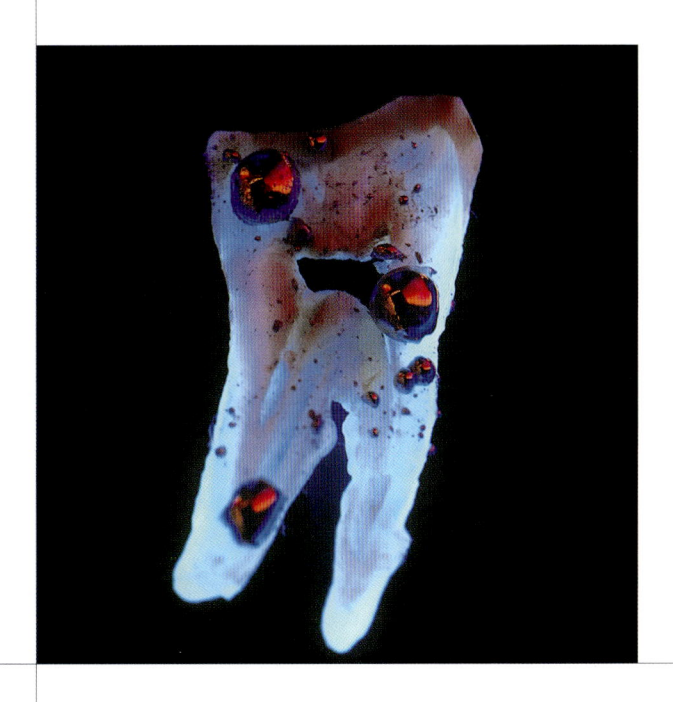

5 Recommended Shade-Matching Protocol

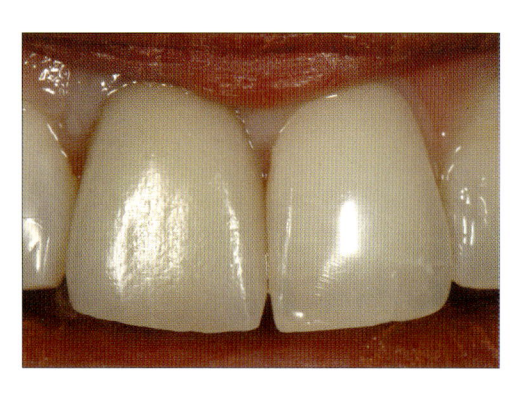

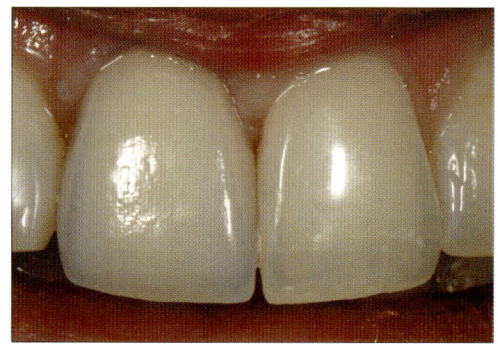

Figs 5-1 and 5-2
Conventional methods of shade selection, when used alone, have several pitfalls, the most significant of which is inaccurate analysis by the clinician. Frequently, multiple restorations are made for the same case, which is an extremely time-consuming and unproductive process. Two crowns were made for the implant abutment at the site of the maxillary right central incisor with an incorrect match: The crown in Fig 5-1 is too opaque and yellowish, and the crown in Fig 5-2 is too low in value (gray).

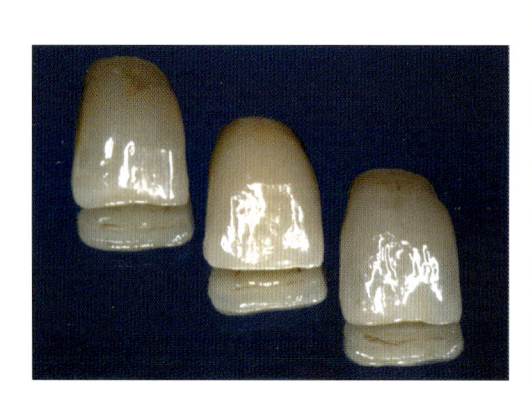

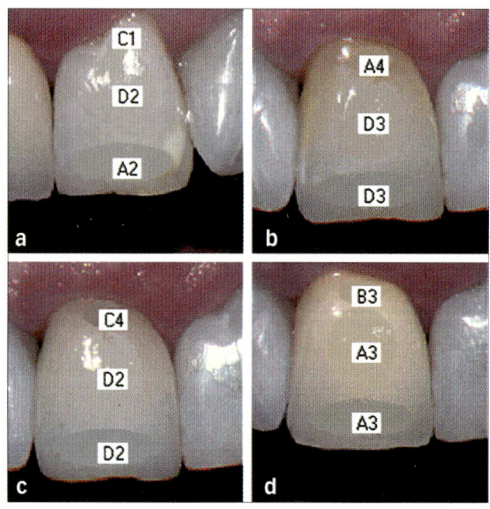

Figs 5-3 and 5-4
Technological shade information also has limitations when used by itself. The three crowns shown in Fig 5-3 were made for the maxillary right central incisor of the same patient without success. The Shade-Vision (X-Rite, Grandville, MI) comparative shade map report in Fig 5-4 shows the discrepancies in shade between the tooth being matched *(a)* and all three restorations *(b to d)*.

The previous two chapters have described the recommended protocols for shade matching using a conventional approach (chapter 3) and a technology-based approach (chapter 4); yet each method, when used by itself, affords limited clinical success. Shade determination using only conventional methodologies often results in failure, frustration, and multiple remakes (Figs 5-1 and 5-2). In addition, although advances in technology have greatly increased the likelihood of a clinically acceptable shade match through accurate shade analysis, shade matching using technological shade systems alone has limitations in the amount of visual information that is provided to the technician (Figs 5-3 and 5-4).

Following much research and clinical evaluation,[1,2] this chapter outlines the authors' recommendations for a more objective and predictable approach to shade matching: a combination of conventional techniques with new technologies.

Seven Steps to a Successful Shade Match

By now the complexity involved in matching a shade is clear. The variables in the operatory and human error are recognized obstacles, and color, being both a science and an art, often can be difficult to gauge. Recognizing that fact, the following case study showcases the best way to take a shade using technology, shade tabs, and reference photography, a combination that will increase esthetic success.

1. Preoperative patient evaluation

The following questions should be considered during the preoperative patient evaluation:

- Are there any contrast effects present that may affect color perception?
- How will the shade selection of one restoration affect the overall smile?
- Is there a significant variance in the shade of the gingival, body, and incisal sections of the teeth?
- Can the patient's teeth be categorized as high in translucency or high in opacity?
- Will material selection significantly affect the final esthetic outcome of the restoration?

Once these questions have been addressed, a treatment plan can be developed, and the clinician can determine the ideal material selection for the case (see chapter 2).

5 Recommended Shade-Matching Protocol

2. Analysis (Figs 5-5 to 5-9)

As outlined in the previous chapters, the best way to analyze the shade is to use all of the tools available. Technology, shade tabs, and reference photographs should all be employed to ascertain the precise shade. First, technology should be used to determine both an overall basic shade as well as shades for each of the three sections of the tooth (gingival, body, and incisal) (Figs 5-5 to 5-9). Shade tabs can then be used to visually confirm the technological shade analysis. In addition, contrasting shade tabs (light and dark) should be used to allow the clinician to better determine and communicate the value of the restoration to the technician.

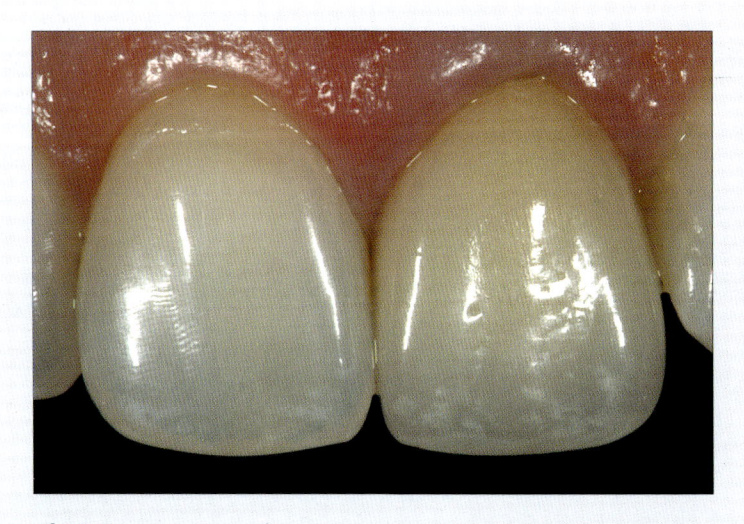

Fig 5-5
Clinical photo of the maxillary central incisors after vital tray bleaching. Twelve years prior to the current treatment, the patient had a post-core foundation restoration and a metal-ceramic crown placed on the left central incisor following root canal treatment. The midfacial gingival margin tissue is starting to develop a slight recession defect, which, along with the poor color match, has caused the patient to seek replacement of the restoration.

SEVEN STEPS TO A SUCCESSFUL SHADE MATCH

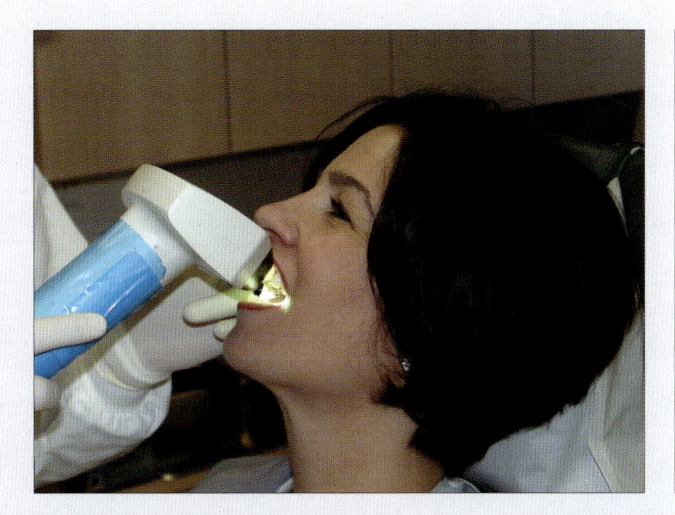

Fig 5-6
SpectroShade (MHT Optic Research, Niederhasli, Switzerland) unit during image capture.

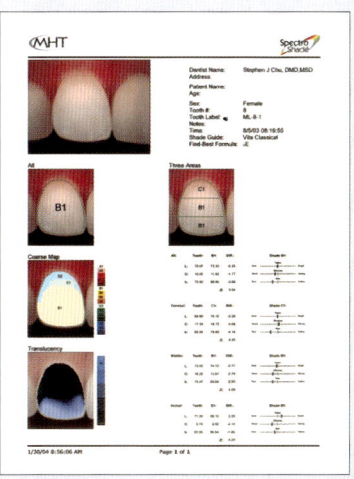

Fig 5-7
SpectroShade comprehensive report for the reference tooth (maxillary right central incisor). Coarse (basic), fine, gingival/body/incisal (GBI), and inferred translucency maps are provided.

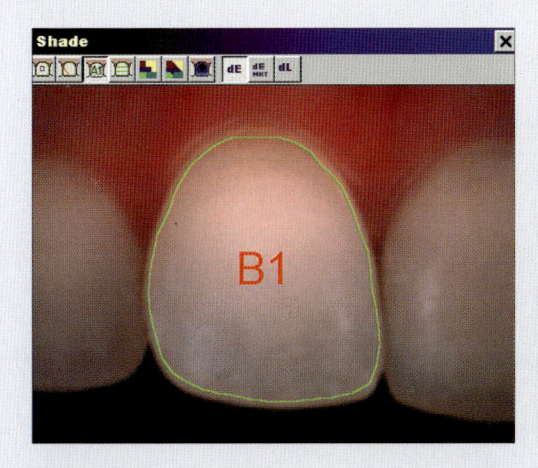

Fig 5-8
A basic Vita B1 shade (Vita, Bad Sackingen, Germany) is found for the reference tooth.

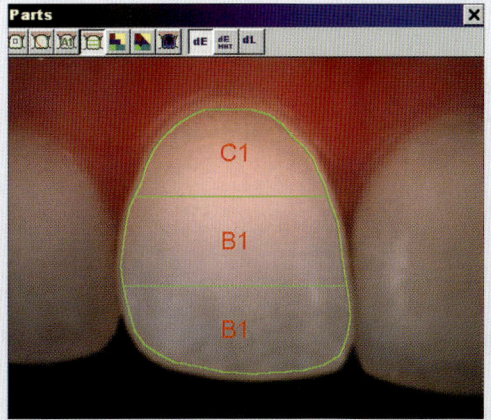

Fig 5-9
GBI shade report shows Vita C1 shade in the gingival third and B1 in the body and incisal thirds of the reference tooth.

5 Recommended Shade-Matching Protocol

3. Communication (Figs 5-10 to 5-15)

The clinician should take reference photographs of the shade tabs suggested by digital analysis (Figs 5-10 to 5-13), as well as the extreme shade tabs (Fig 5-14) next to the dentition to be matched. In addition, reference photographs showing the full smile and the shade of the surrounding dentition should be taken. It is important to remember to take such photographs from varying angles and under different lighting conditions to best capture the subtleties of the tooth shade and texture (Fig 5-15; see also Figs 5-11 to 5-13).

An 18% reflectance gray card should be used as a background in reference photography to eliminate extraneous color distractions and contrast effects (see chapter 2).

Once the shade information is gathered by the clinician, it must be delivered to the lab. The technology-based analysis can be delivered electronically. Reference photographs and written descriptions, critical pieces of information for accurate shade communication, may be sent to the laboratory as hard copies or as electronic files by e-mail or on CD.

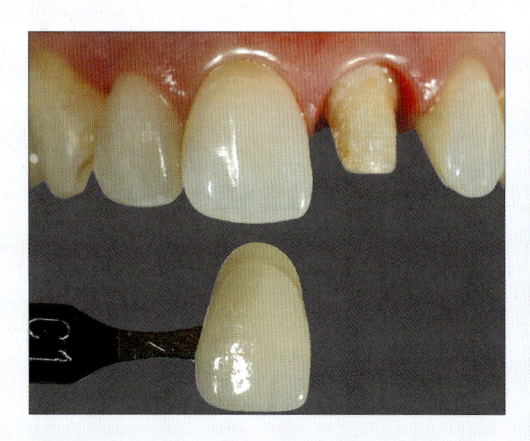

Fig 5-10
Shade tabs are used to visually confirm the findings of the technology-based shade analysis reports. Here, Vitapan shade C1 (Vita) is referenced based on the gingival shade found by the SpectroShade system. The shade tabs were photographed using twin spot flash from the sides.

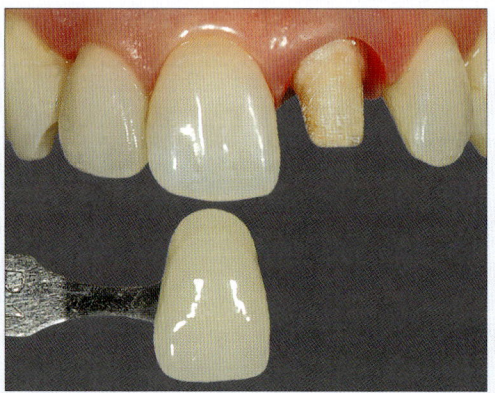

Fig 5-11
Vitapan B1 shade tab with twin flash from the sides.

Seven Steps to a Successful Shade Match

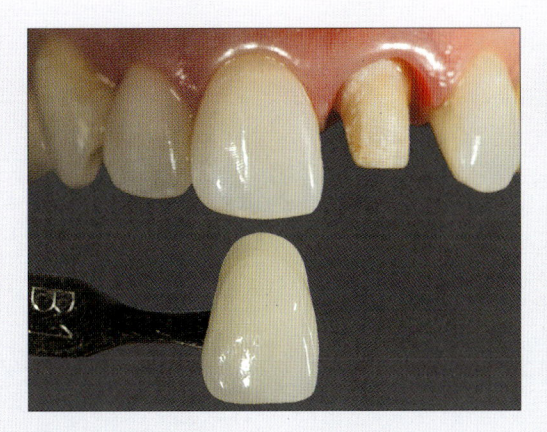

Fig 5-12
Vitapan B1 shade tab with flash from the top.

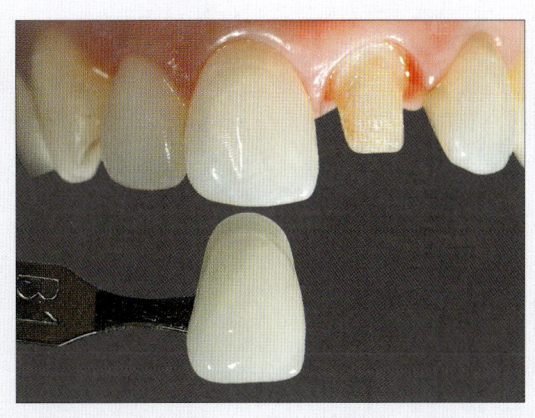

Fig 5-13
Vitapan B1 shade tab with flash from the bottom. Note the change in visual shade comparison when flash orientation is changed (Figs 5-11 to 5-13).

Fig 5-14
Composite photograph with extreme shade tabs to assess value change. *(left to right)* Chromascop bleached shade 010 (Ivoclar-Vivadent, Amherst, NY), Vitapan B1, and Vitapan B4.

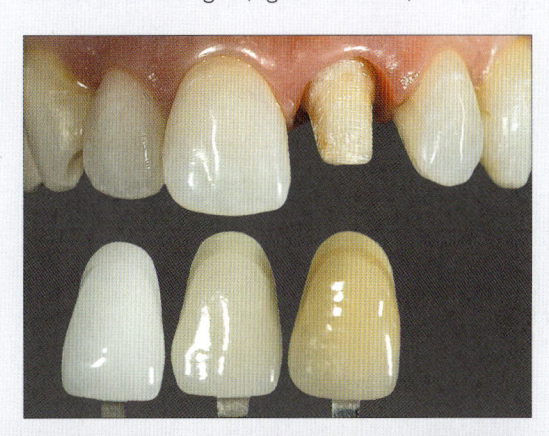

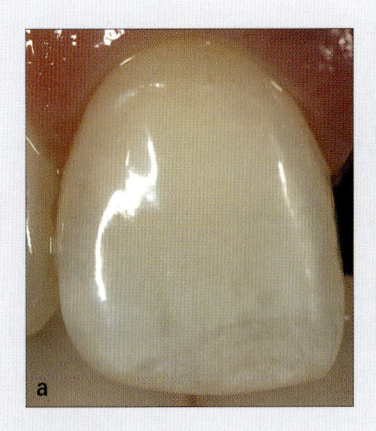

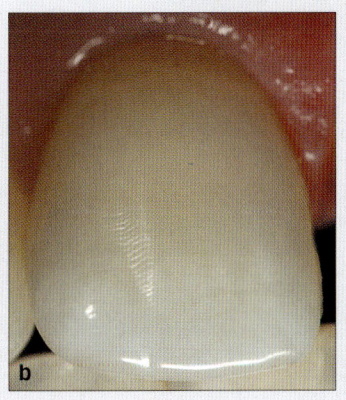

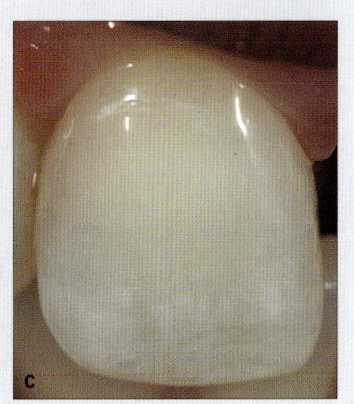

Fig 5-15
Photographs of the maxillary right central incisor (reference tooth) with lighting from the side *(a)*, the bottom *(b)*, and the top *(c)*, showing nuances in tooth shade and characterization.

5 Recommended Shade-Matching Protocol

4. Interpretation (Figs 5-16 to 5-18)

The laboratory must interpret all of the pieces of shade information provided. The reference photographs help the lab technician to better understand the shade tab selection and the variance in value and chroma, while the digital color map provides a detailed depiction of the shade reading. The technician translates this information into the language of the ceramic system to be used, creating maps of where the ceramic system's special effects powders should be used to achieve the desired nuances in shade (Figs 5-16 to 5-18).

Most technicians are familiar with the various nomenclatures and effects of different porcelain systems. This knowledge allows them to select the best ceramic system for the esthetic restorative needs of each clinical case.

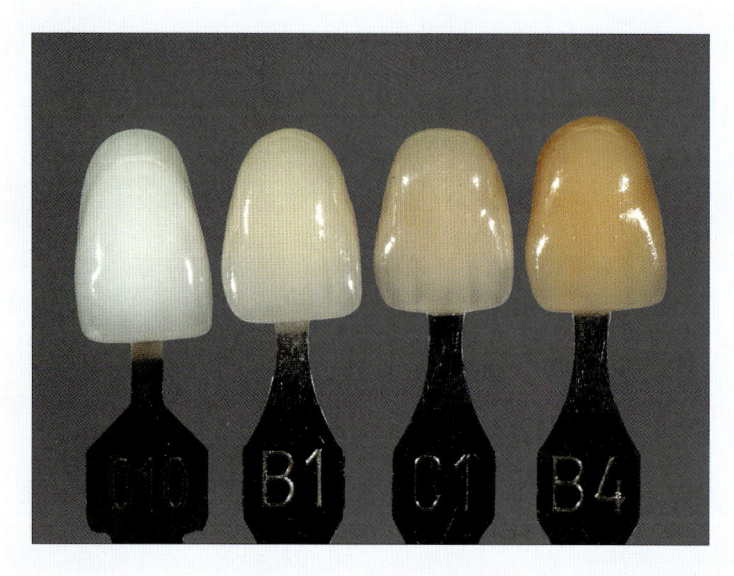

Fig 5-16
An 18% reflectance gray card is also used in the dental laboratory by the technician to assess the value differences in shade tabs seen in the reference photographs.

SEVEN STEPS TO A SUCCESSFUL SHADE MATCH

Fig 5-17
Shade tab information is interpreted and converted into the language and nomenclature of the ceramic system used.

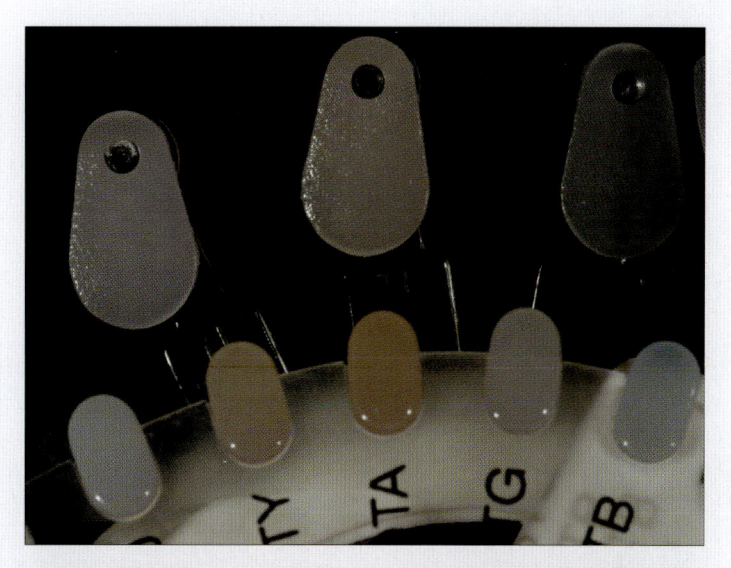

Fig 5-18
The language of the ceramic system is transposed onto a printout of a clinical photograph to create a special effects color location and distribution map.

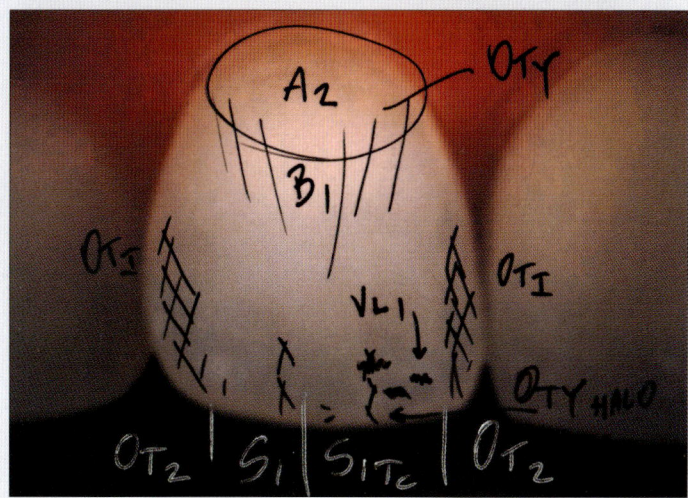

5 Recommended Shade-Matching Protocol

5. Fabrication (Figs 5-19 to 5-29)

After assessing the shade and determining what material works best given the particular clinical application, the lab technician fabricates the restoration and adds the necessary details in the staining and glazing stage to match the opposing dentition (Figs 5-19 to 5-29).

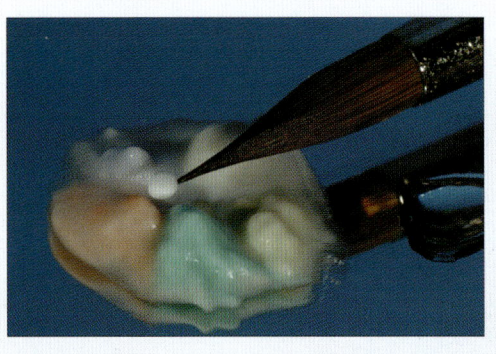

Fig 5-19
Ceramic powders are selected and mixed to a creamy consistency with modeling fluid.

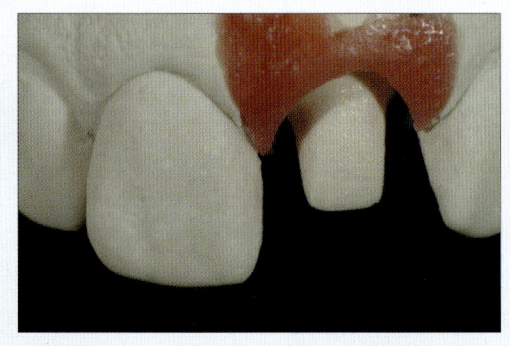

Fig 5-20
A refractory cast with simulated soft tissue is fabricated for buildup of an all-ceramic crown.

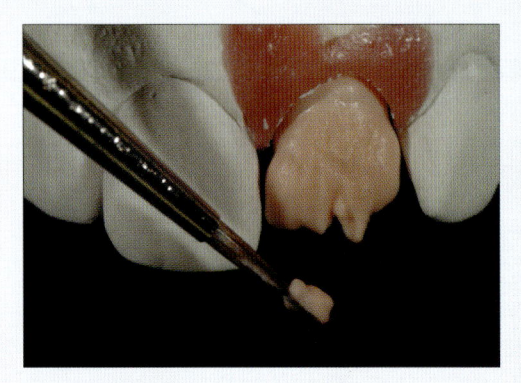

Fig 5-21
Secondary dentin is layered at the cervical area, then dentin is layered on top and blended toward the body and incisal areas.

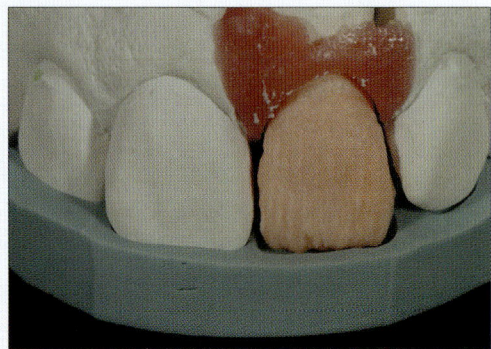

Fig 5-22
An incisal matrix is used in the dentinal ceramic buildup to guide the vertical and horizontal incisal edge positions.

110

SEVEN STEPS TO A SUCCESSFUL SHADE MATCH

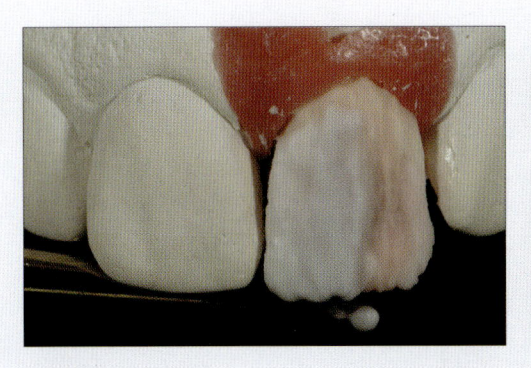

Fig 5-23
Dentin ceramic material is layered with incisal enamel and special effects (opal transparent) powders.

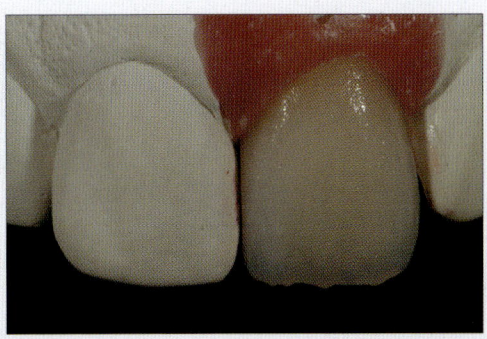

Fig 5-24
Crown after completion of first bisque bake.

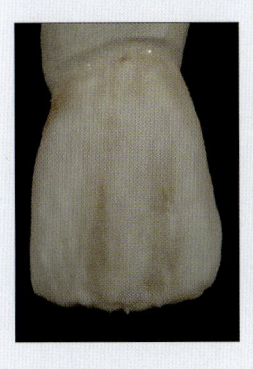

Fig 5-25
Second ceramic buildup with opal transparent powders (HeraCeram [Heraeus-Kulzer-Jelenko, Armonk, NY]).

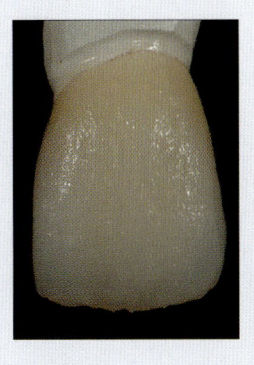

Fig 5-26
Crown after second bisque bake with opalescent powders.

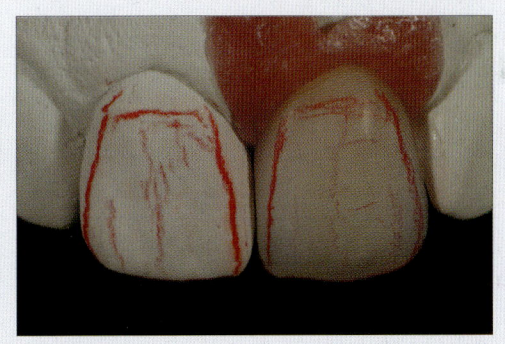

Fig 5-27
Final shaping of restoration with a red wax-based pencil. A lead-based pencil should not be used because the lead dust can contaminate and discolor the porcelain.

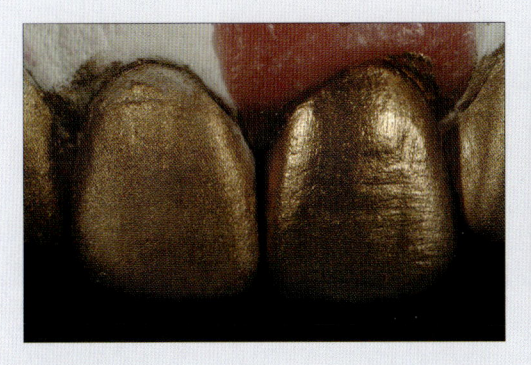

Fig 5-28
Gold powder is used to visualize the surface texture of the restoration.

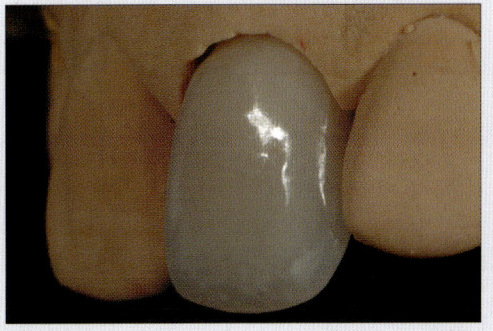

Fig 5-29
The restoration is glazed for characterization and polished to give the proper surface luster.

5 Recommended Shade-Matching Protocol

6. Verification (Figs 5-30 to 5-35)

The shade is verified using both conventional and technological methods (Figs 5-30 to 5-35). If the restoration does not match, extrinsic colorants are used to adjust the shade, then the virtual try-in and shade tab comparisons are repeated. Once accuracy is confirmed, the restoration is sent back to the clinician.

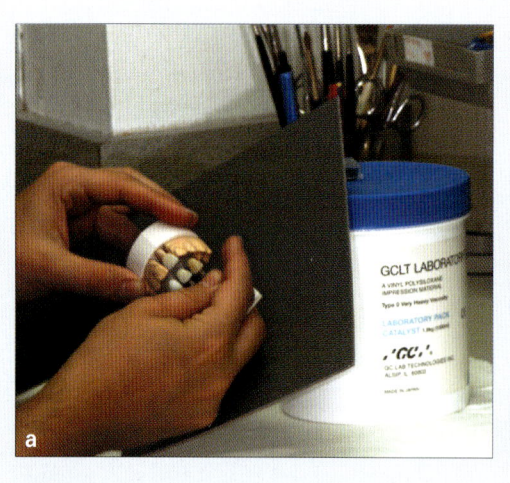

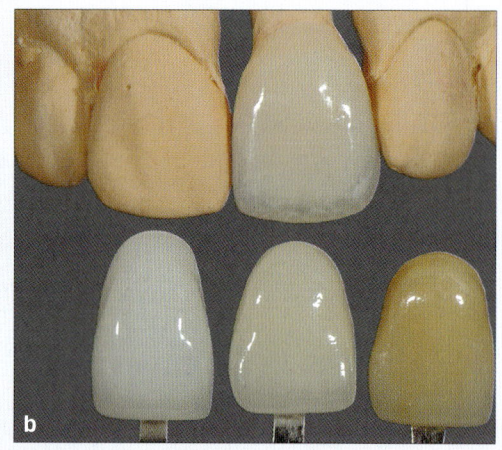

Fig 5-30
(a) The extreme shade tabs used in the reference photographs are compared to the completed restoration against the 18% gray card. *(b)* Close-up of the extreme shade tabs being compared to the restoration.

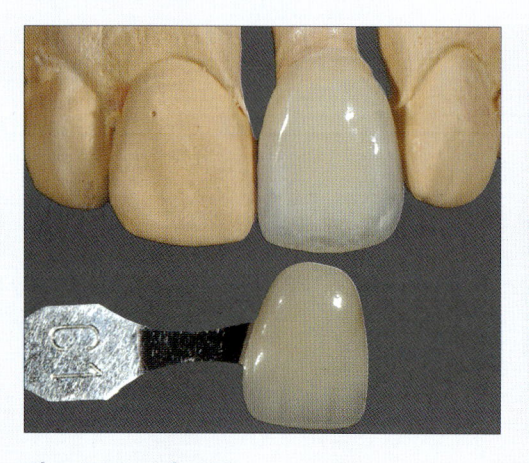

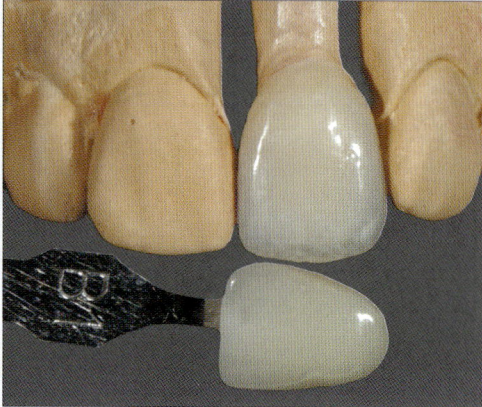

Figs 5-31 and 5-32
Shades C1 (Fig 5-31) and B1 (Fig 5-32) (used in the reference photographs) are also compared to the completed restoration against the 18% gray card.

Seven Steps to a Successful Shade Match

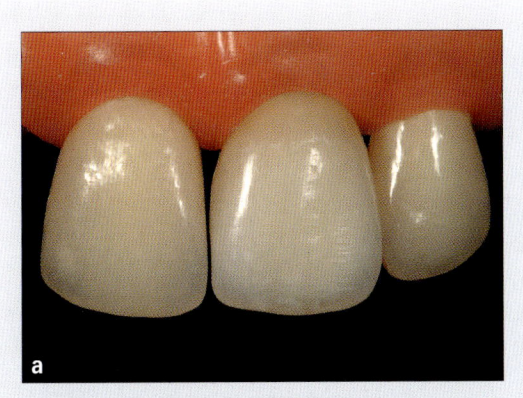

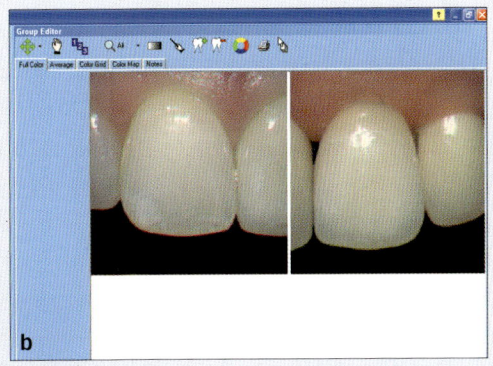

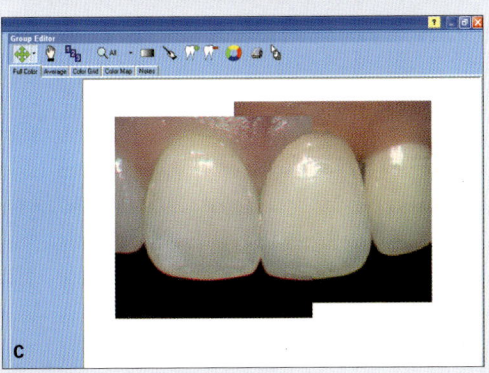

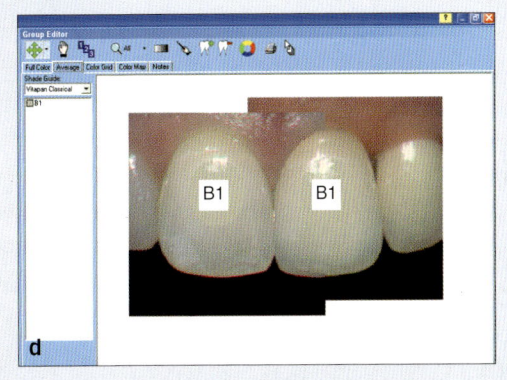

Fig 5-33

ShadeVision virtual try-in. *(a)* The crown is placed in the restoration holder for scanning. *(b)* Image of the natural right central incisor and scan of the crown for left central incisor. *(c)* The virtual try-in confirms a visual match. *(d)* The report verifies a base shade of B1.

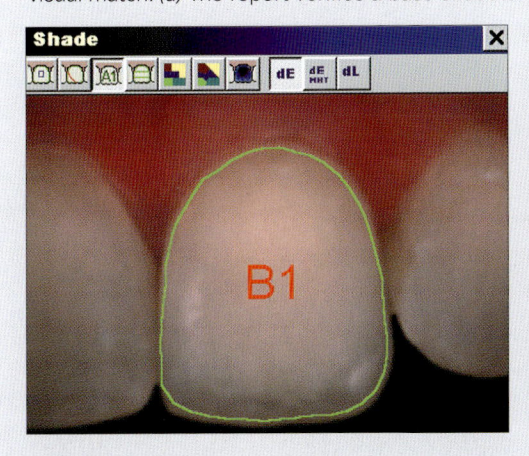

Fig 5-34

SpectroShade verification using spectrophotometric analysis. Shade B1 is again confirmed.

Fig 5-35

GBI shade distribution map verifies a close match, although there is a slight shade discrepancy at the gingival third (D2 versus C1 [see Fig 5-9]). However, there is a very small ΔE between shades C1 and D2.

5 Recommended Shade-Matching Protocol

7. Placement (Figs 5-36 to 5-44)

The ultimate verification of the restoration's accuracy occurs when the clinician places the restoration (Figs 5-36 to 5-44). If the restoration does not match, it will be immediately evident. Using this protocol (steps 1 to 6) should minimize if not eliminate the need for remakes at this clinical try-in stage. If, however, a remake or color adjustment is required, the analysis should be repeated and new reference photographs taken with the new restoration in place. Such problems are usually caused by errors in analysis, communication, or both.

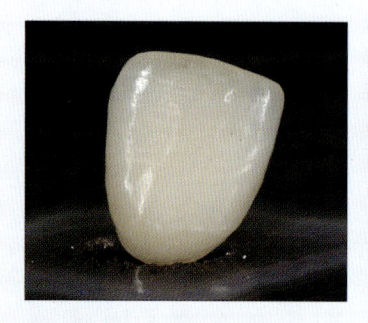

Fig 5-36 The all-ceramic crown is prepared for cementation with resin composite cement (hydrofluoric acid etch, silane air dry, and bonding resin).

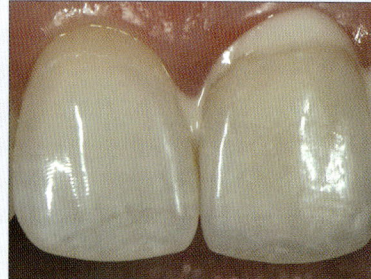

Fig 5-37 The restoration is placed with a trial cement to visually verify the shade intraorally.

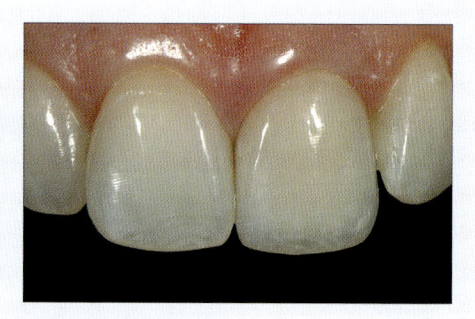

Fig 5-38 Close-up intraoral view of cemented all-ceramic crown on the left central incisor.

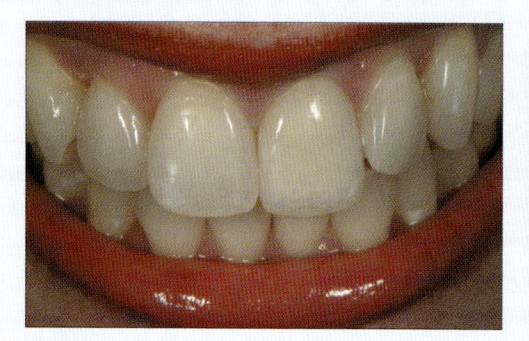

Fig 5-39 Close-up of smile with crown in place.

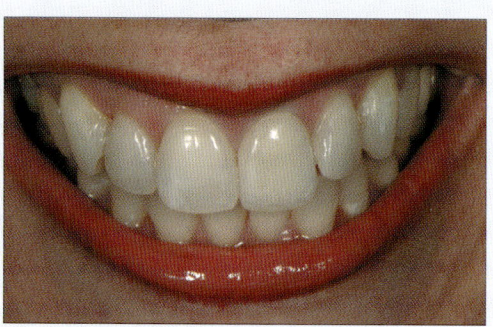

Fig 5-40 Full view of smile.

SEVEN STEPS TO A SUCCESSFUL SHADE MATCH

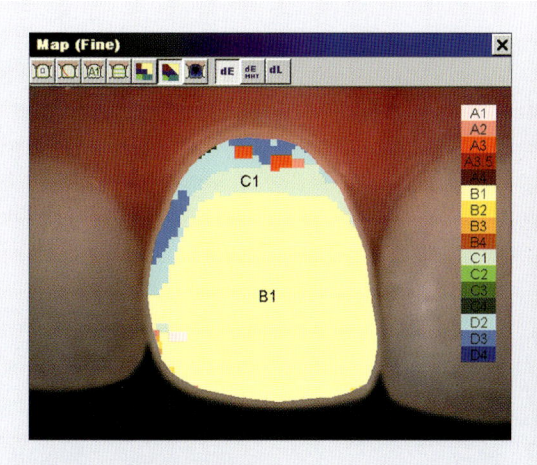

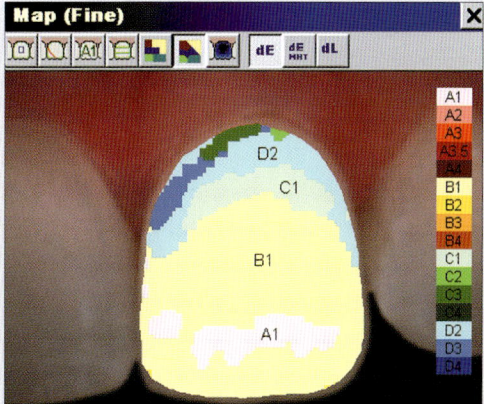

Figs 5-41 and 5-42
Fine shade maps (SpectroShade) of the natural right central incisor (Fig 5-41) and the all-ceramic crown on the left central incisor (Fig 5-42). A close shade match is confirmed.

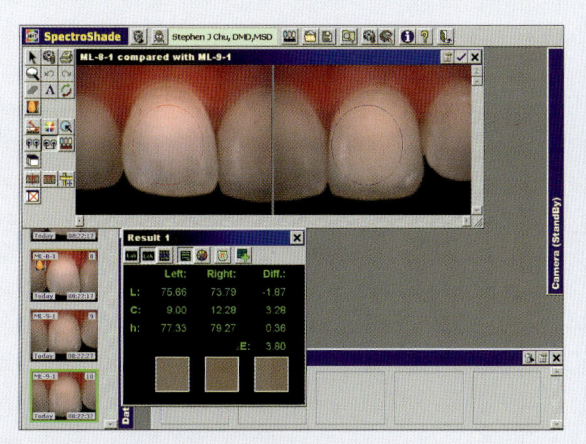

Fig 5-43
Total ΔE of the natural right central incisor compared to the crown on the left central incisor is 3.80. The value ΔE is −1.87. A ΔE for value of less than 2.0 is highly clinically acceptable.

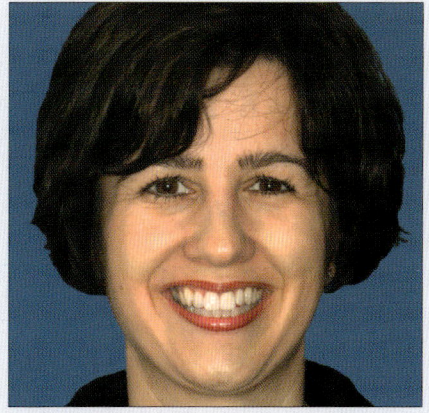

Fig 5-44
Full-face clinical photograph. The patient is pleased with the final esthetic restorative outcome. With this recommended shade-taking protocol, challenging anterior restorations can be matched predictably with a clinically acceptable result in one visit.

115

5 Recommended Shade-Matching Protocol

Summary

- Successful shade taking involves a combination of technology, shade tabs, and reference photography.
- Details added by the lab technician in the fabrication process can often increase the natural appearance of a shade.
- Technology-based systems are extremely useful in the analysis and verification of a shade match.

References

1. Chu SJ. Use of a reflectance spectrophotometer in evaluating shade change resulting from tooth-whitening products. J Esthet Dent 2003;15(suppl 1):S42–S48.
2. Devigus A. Die digitale Farbmessung in der Zahnmedizin. Quintessenz 2003;54:495–500.

Appendix: Clinical Cases

Includes shade-matching protocol for:

- Single anterior all-ceramic (Procera) crown
- Single anterior all-ceramic (In-Ceram) crown
- Single anterior implant-supported metal-ceramic crown
- Single anterior ceramic laminate veneer
- Two anterior all-ceramic crowns
- Two anterior all-ceramic crowns with one anterior metal-ceramic crown
- Four anterior ceramic laminate veneers
- Single posterior all-ceramic crown
- Ten ceramic laminate veneers to match bleached teeth
- Two anterior direct composite restorations

The following clinical cases demonstrate the use of the shade-matching protocol presented in chapter 5, ie, a combination of conventional and technology-based techniques. If this approach is followed, it is nearly assured that an accurate shade match will be achieved the first time, eliminating the need for any remakes.

APPENDIX: CLINICAL CASES

Case 1: Single Anterior All-Ceramic (Procera) Crown

A 68-year-old woman was in need of a full-coverage restoration on her maxillary right central incisor (Fig C1-1). The existing metal-ceramic crown had been fabricated 5 years before the current treatment, and the cement bond on the post-core foundation restoration had failed (Fig C1-2). A bonded post-core system was used to reconstruct the lost coronal tooth structure (Fig C1-3). Two types of technology-based systems were used for shade analysis: ShadeScan (Cynovad, Montreal, Canada) (Fig C1-4) and SpectroShade (MHT Optic Research, Niederhasli, Switzerland) (Figs C1-5 and C1-6). There was agreement between the two systems that the base shade should be Vitapan D2. Reference photographs were taken to communicate shade more effectively. Shade D2 (Fig C1-7) and A2 (Fig C1-8) were referenced as the matching shades, and shade A3 (Fig C1-9) and A1 (Fig C1-10) were extreme shade references for value and chroma interpretation. A gypsum die model was fabricated, and a Procera semi-translucent coping (Nobel Biocare, Fairlawn, NJ) (Fig C1-11) was selected as the restorative material that would best suit the esthetic and functional needs of the case. The ceramic buildup was made using Creation AV porcelain (Jensen Industries, New Haven, CT) (Figs C1-12 to C1-17). The crown was placed with clinical success (Figs C1-18 to C1-20).

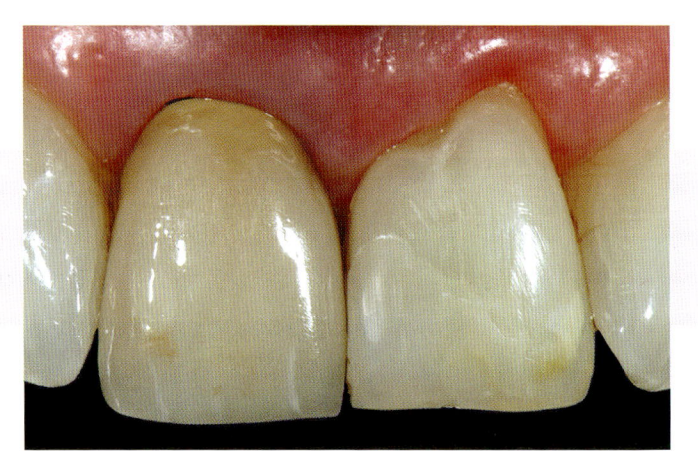

Fig C1-1

Case 1: Single Anterior All-Ceramic (Procera) Crown

Fig C1-2

Fig C1-3

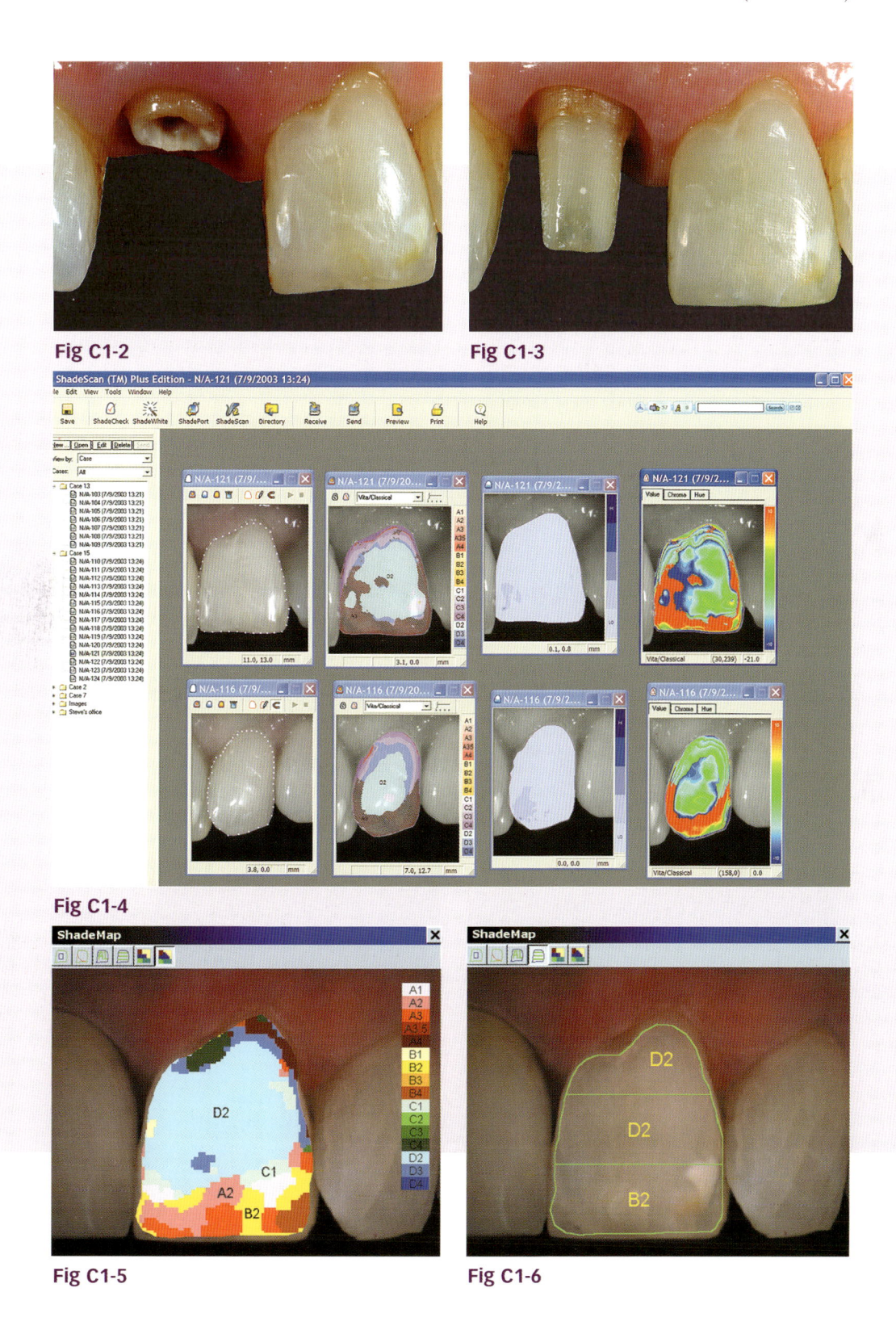

Fig C1-4

Fig C1-5

Fig C1-6

119

Appendix: Clinical Cases

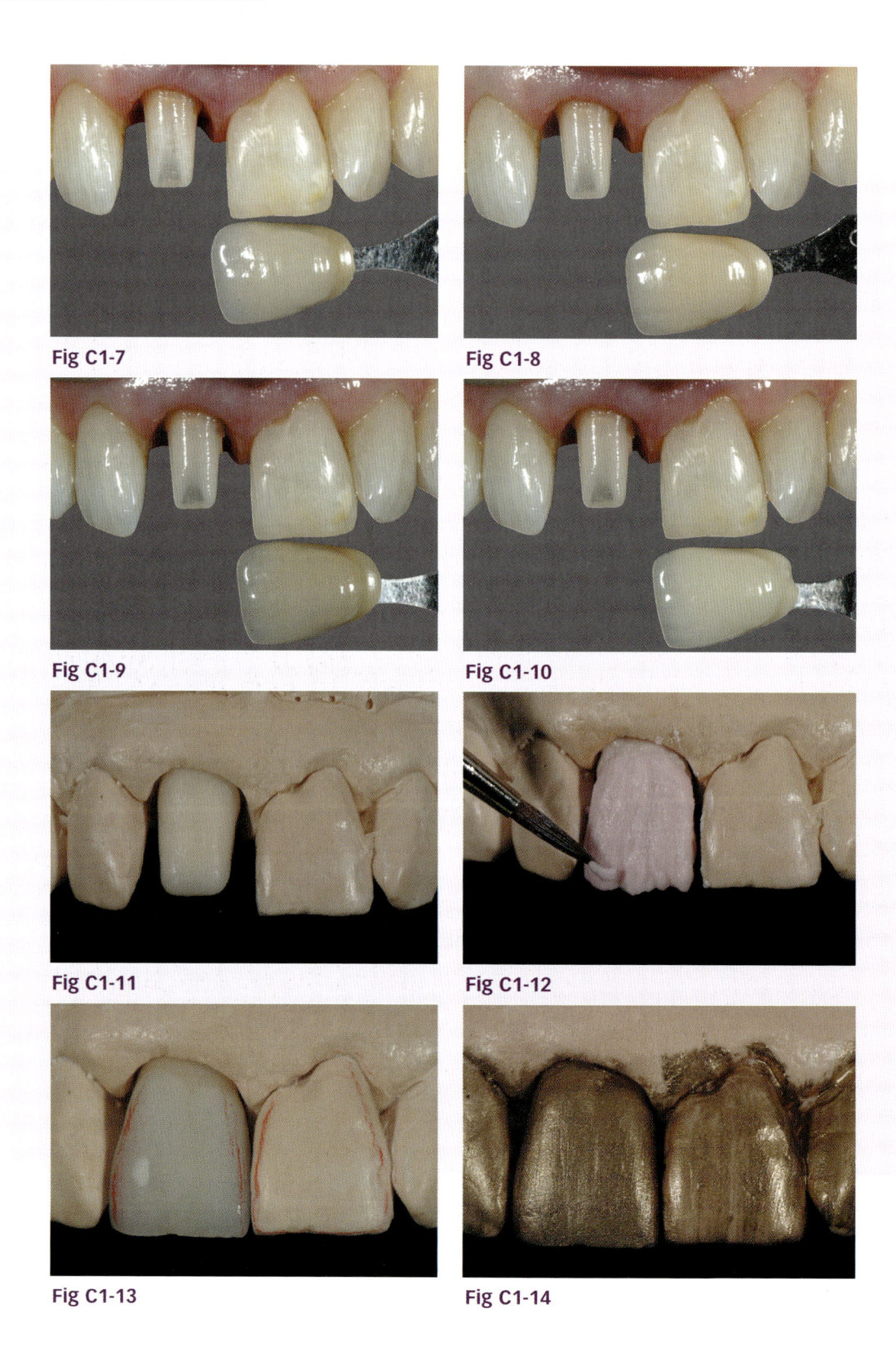

Fig C1-7

Fig C1-8

Fig C1-9

Fig C1-10

Fig C1-11

Fig C1-12

Fig C1-13

Fig C1-14

Case 1: Single Anterior All-Ceramic (Procera) Crown

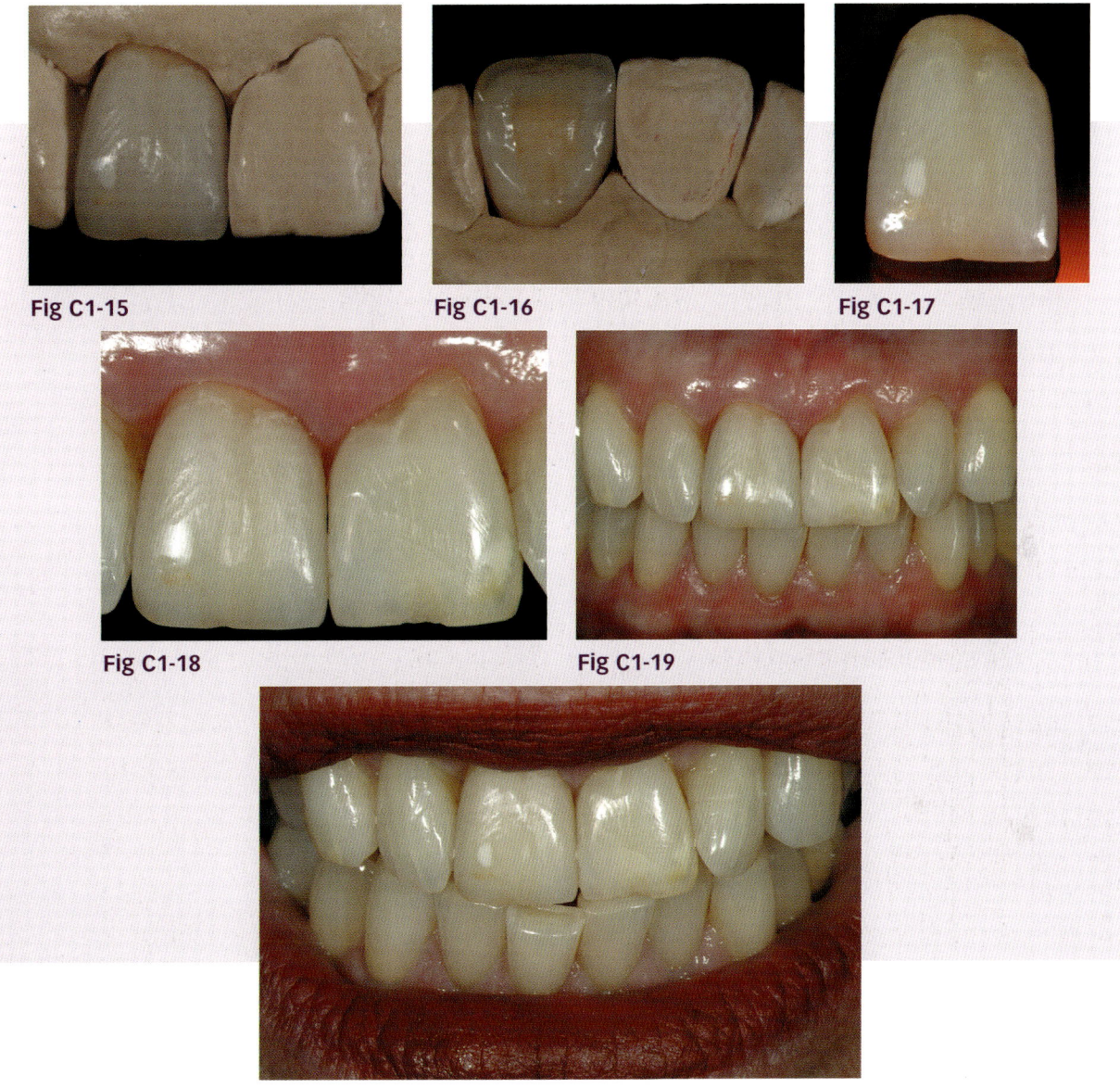

Fig C1-15

Fig C1-16

Fig C1-17

Fig C1-18

Fig C1-19

Fig C1-20

121

Appendix: Clinical Cases

Case 2: Single Anterior All-Ceramic (In-Ceram) Crown

A 55-year-old woman presented with a broken all-ceramic crown on her maxillary right central incisor (Fig C2-1). The tooth was nonvital as a result of root canal treatment. Radiographs were taken and a provisional crown was fabricated as an emergency treatment. During the following appointment, the preparation was completed (Fig C2-2), and impressions of both arches were made using a polyether impression material. Technology-based shade analysis (SpectroShade [MHT Optic Research, Niederhasli, Switzerland]) (Fig C2-3) and digital photography were used in this case for color and form communication with the lab technician. Shade analysis was performed on the left central incisor prior to preparation (Fig C2-4).

A new full-ceramic crown (In-Ceram [Vita, Bad Sackingen, Germany]) was fabricated on the right central incisor using CAD/CAM technology. The appropriate ceramic materials (Vita VM9) were layered and fired to maturation. Prior to cementation, the shade of the fabricated crown was verified with the SpectroShade device (Fig C2-5). Final comparative SpectroShade analysis showed an overall ΔE of less than 1.5 and a value ΔE of less than 1 (Fig C2-6). This means that the difference in shade between the restoration and the adjacent tooth is not visible with the human eye. A successful esthetic result was achieved with a single fabrication (Figs C2-7 and C2-8).

Laboratory work by Giordano Lombardi, CDT, Zurich, Switzerland.

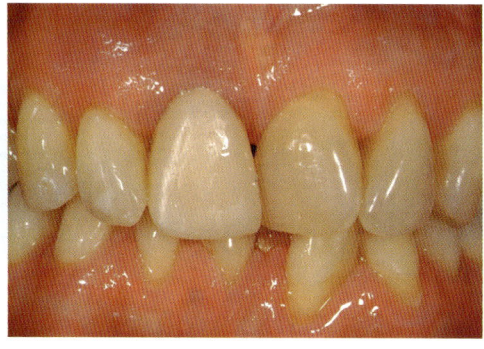

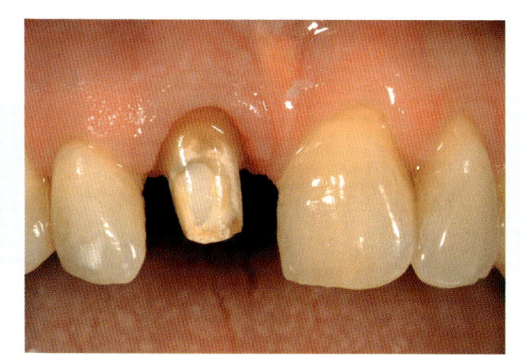

Fig C2-1

Fig C2-2

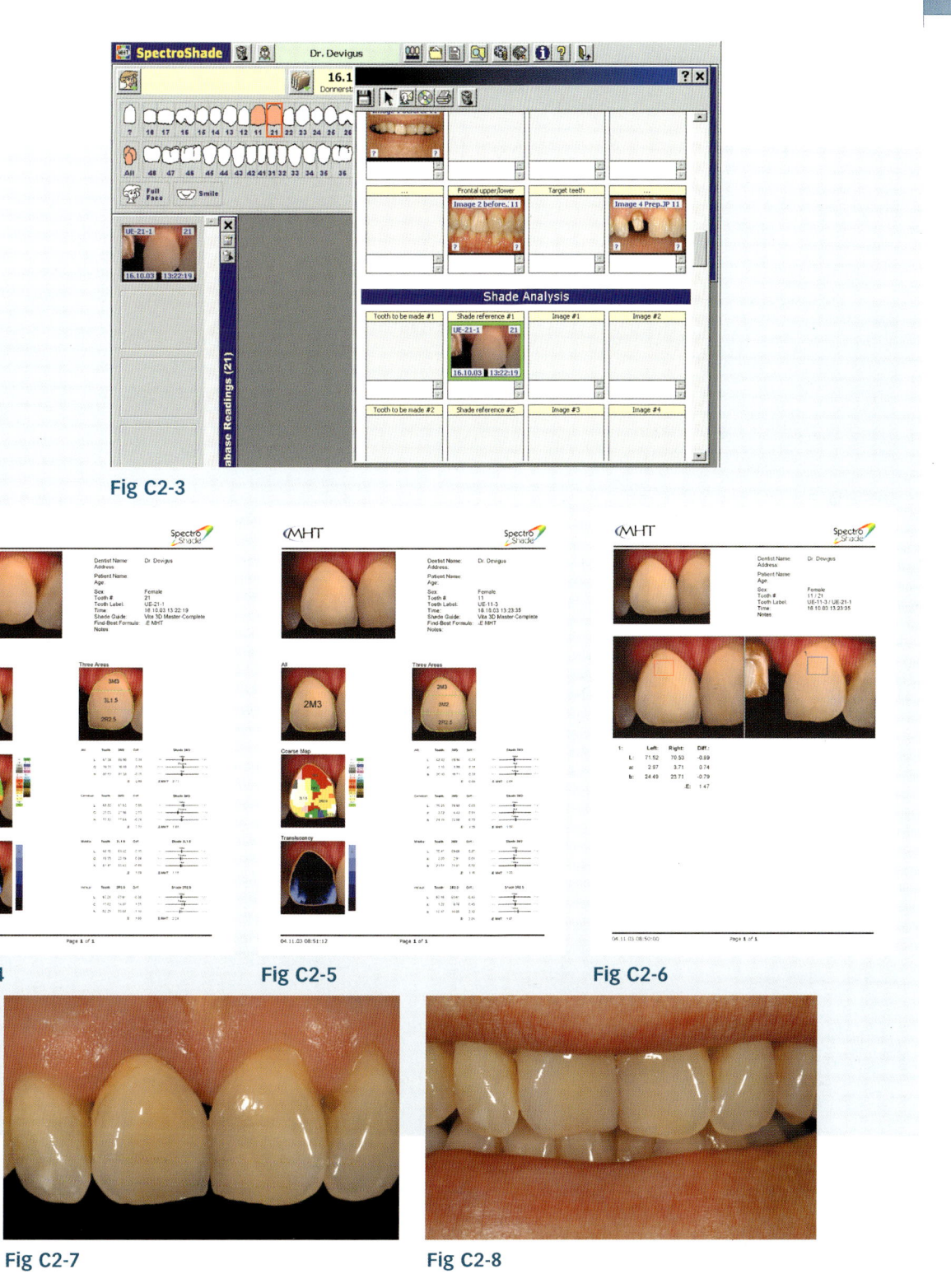

CASE 2: SINGLE ANTERIOR ALL-CERAMIC (IN-CERAM) CROWN

Fig C2-3

Fig C2-4

Fig C2-5

Fig C2-6

Fig C2-7

Fig C2-8

123

APPENDIX: CLINICAL CASES

Case 3: Single Anterior Implant-Supported Metal-Ceramic Crown

A 54-year-old man presented with a dental history of failing root canal treatment on the maxillary right central incisor (Fig C3-1). A bone allograft (Puros [Tutogen Medical, Allachua, FL]) was placed (Fig C3-2) following atraumatic surgical removal, and a selected surface implant (Osseotite [3i, Palm Beach Gardens, FL]) was placed 6 months after socket maturation (Fig C3-3). A custom implant abutment was inserted (Fig C3-4), and several metal-ceramic crowns were made for the right central incisor using only conventional shade determination with poor esthetic results (Fig C3-5).

The recommended shade protocol, employing technology-based shade analysis (SpectroShade [MHT Optic Research, Niederhasli, Switzerland]) (Figs C3-6 to C3-9) and reference photographs for color communication and value assessment (Figs C3-10 to C3-12), was then used to fabricate a new metal-ceramic crown. A metal alloy coping was waxed, cast, and finished, and opaque porcelain was applied (Fig C3-13). The appropriate ceramic materials were layered (Fig C3-14) and fired to maturation. Surface texture was verified using gold powder (Fig C3-15), and the restoration was glazed and polished (Fig C3-16). The final comparative SpectroShade analysis showed an overall ΔE of 3.65 and a ΔL (value) of less than 2.0 (Fig C3-17). The value parameter is the most signficant because the human eye can perceive differences in the lightness and darkness of shades more easily than it can detect variations in hue. A successful esthetic result was achieved in one attempt using the recommended shade-matching protocol (Fig C3-18).

Surgical and restorative portions of this case performed by Drs Dennis Tarnow and Marion Brown (New York, New York), respectively.

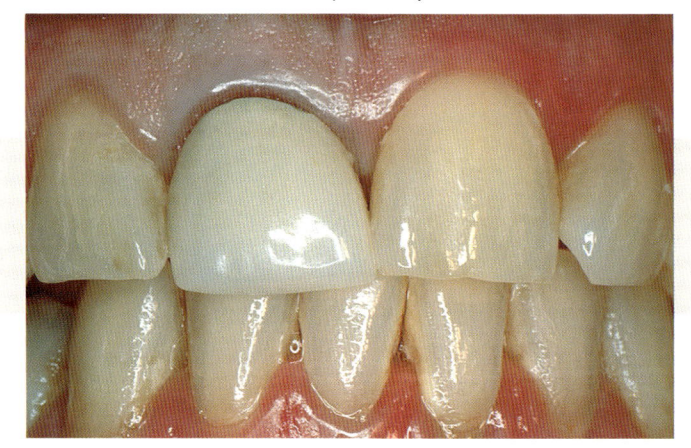

Fig C3-1

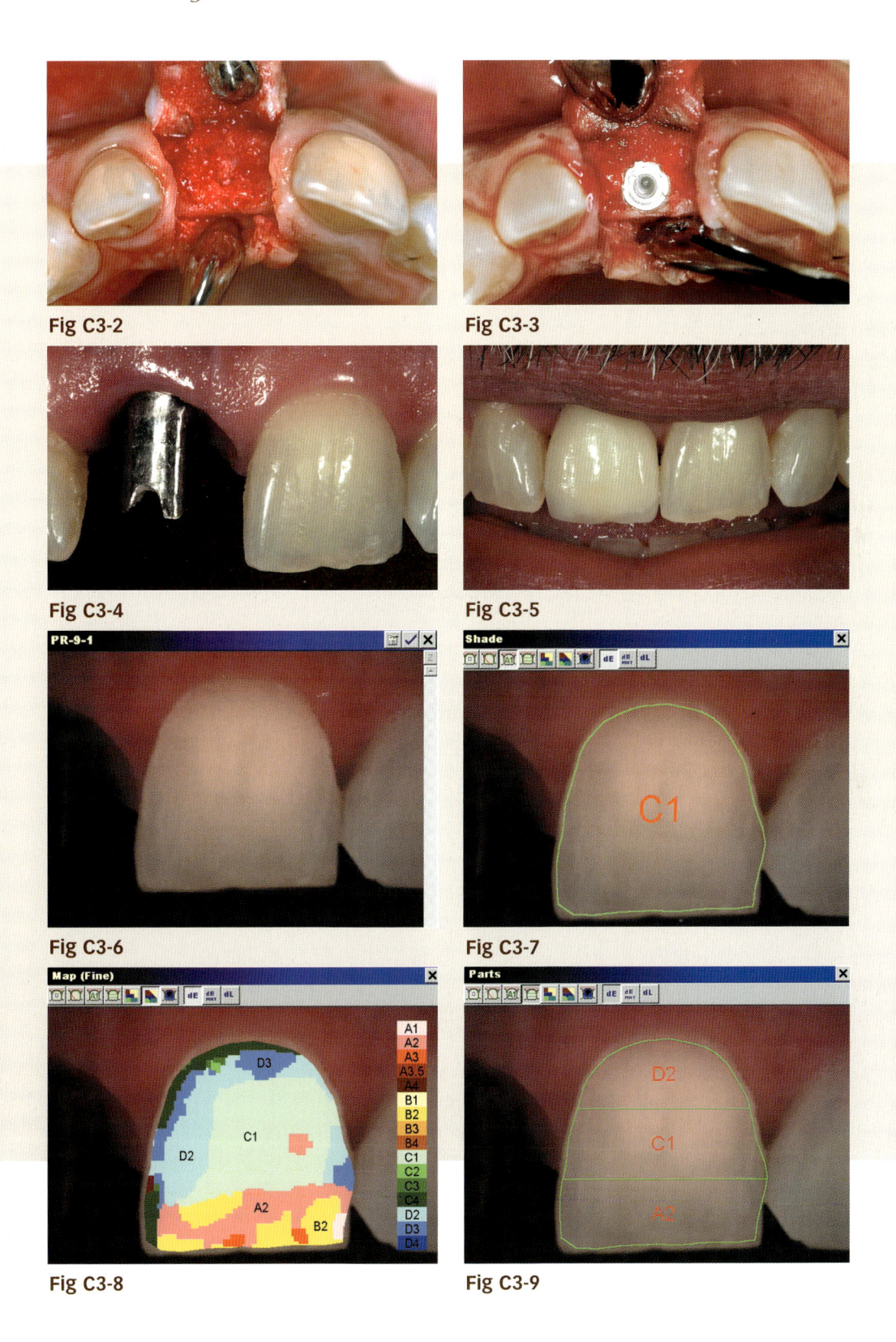

Case 3: Single Anterior Implant-Supported Metal-Ceramic Crown

Fig C3-2

Fig C3-3

Fig C3-4

Fig C3-5

Fig C3-6

Fig C3-7

Fig C3-8

Fig C3-9

125

Appendix: Clinical Cases

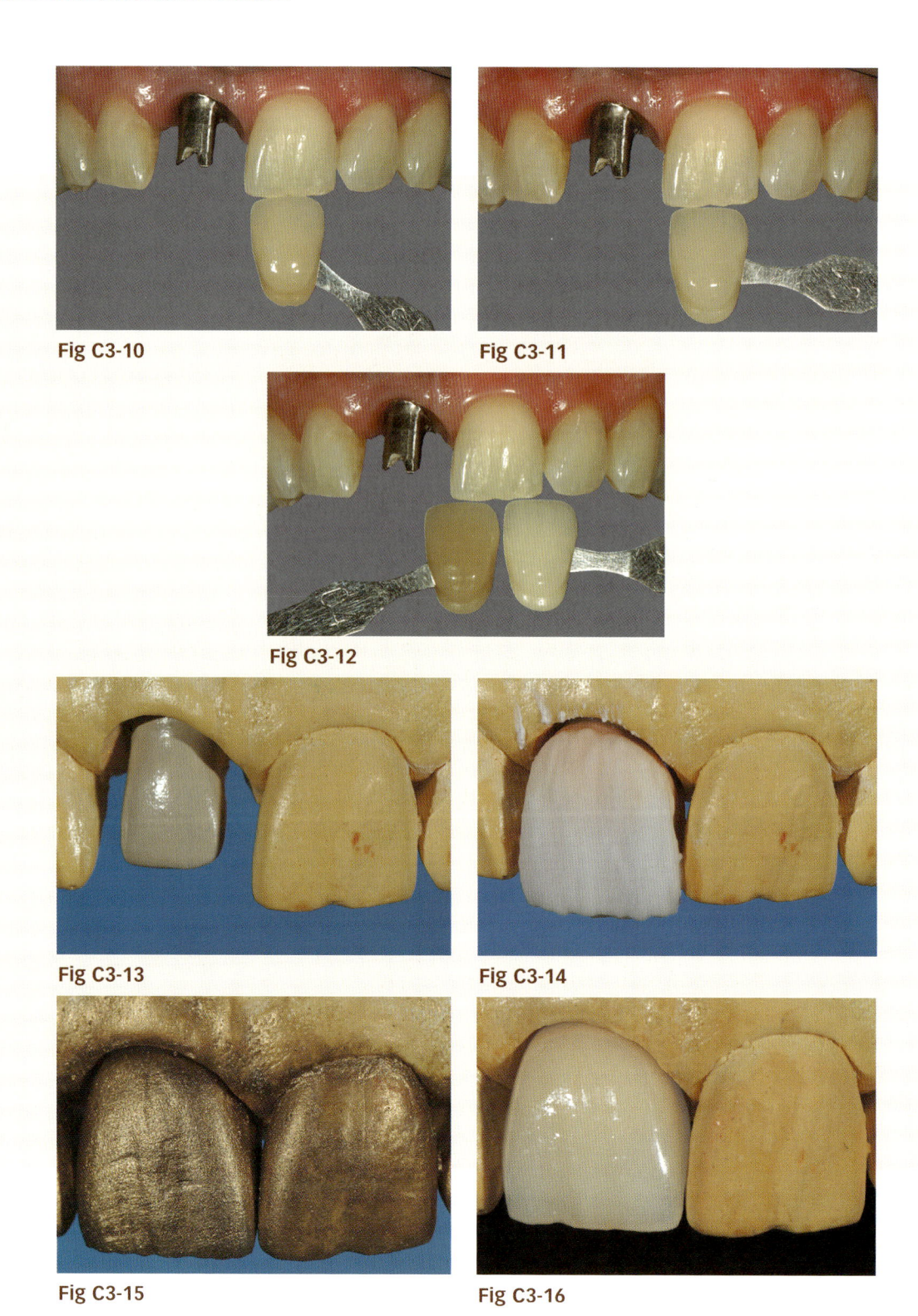

Fig C3-10

Fig C3-11

Fig C3-12

Fig C3-13

Fig C3-14

Fig C3-15

Fig C3-16

126

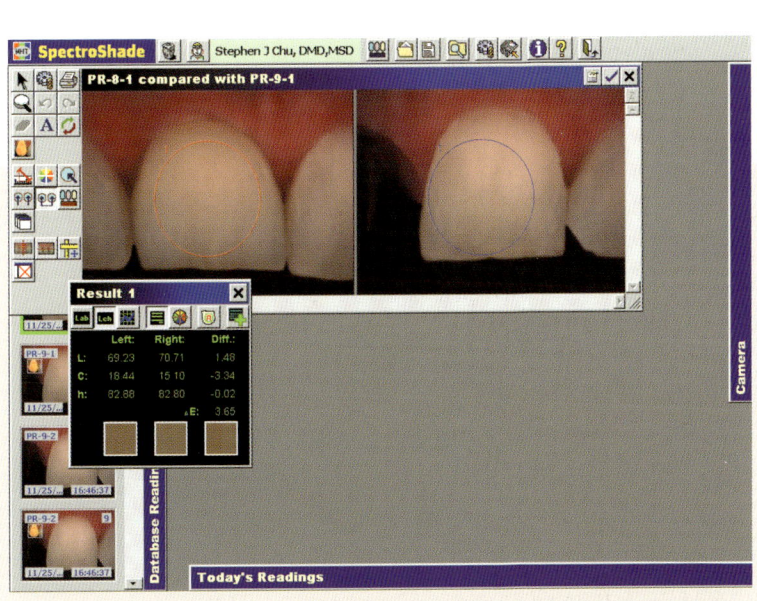

Case 3: Single Anterior Implant-Supported Metal-Ceramic Crown

Fig C3-17

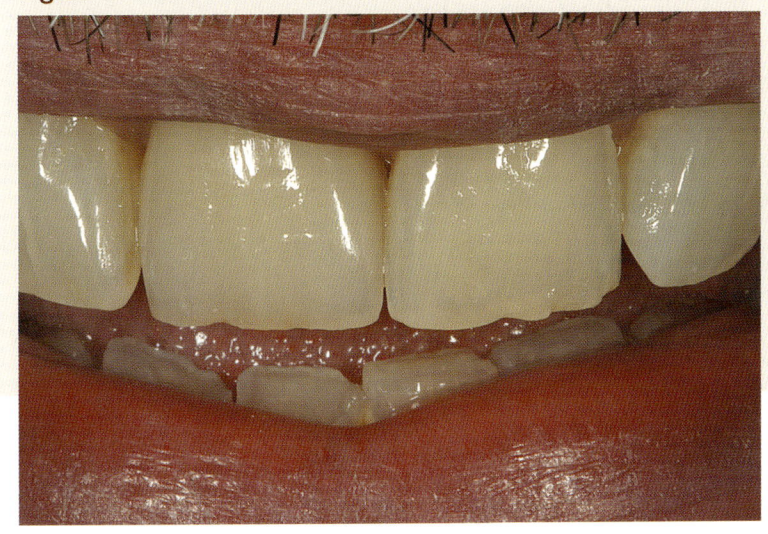

Fig C3-18

Case 4: Single Anterior Ceramic Laminate Veneer

A 79-year-old woman presented with significant interproximal mesial and distal decay on her maxillary left central incisor (Figs C4-1 and C4-2). Because of the high translucency of the tooth to be matched, a ceramic laminate veneer was the restoration of choice. ShadeScan (Cynovad, Montreal, Canada) (Fig C4-3), ShadeVision (X-Rite, Grandville, MI) (Fig C4-4), and SpectroShade (MHT Optic Research, Niederhasli, Switzerland) (Fig C4-5) were used for shade analysis of the reference tooth. Vitapan A4 (Fig C4-6), C3 (Fig C4-7), and A3.5 (Fig C4-8) shade tabs (Vita, Bad Sackingen, Germany) were used in the reference photographs based on the SpectroShade GBI map (see Fig C4-5). In addition, reference photographs of extreme shade tabs were taken for value determination; a Vitapan C4 tab was selected for the dark reference (Fig C4-9) and an A2 for the light reference (Fig C4-10).

Mesial and distal decay were removed, and the shade of the remaining natural tooth material was determined to be A3.5 (Fig C4-11). A paste deflection tissue management system (Expa-syl [Kerr, Orange, CA]) was used to control crevicular fluids and expose the apical extent of the preparation margin (Fig C4-12) prior to final impression making with a polyvinyl siloxane material (Honigum [Zenith/DMG, Englewood, NJ]) (Fig C4-13). A gypsum cast was poured and duplicated for a refractory cast (Fig C4-14). An incisal addition silicone index was used during the dentin ceramic buildup to establish the incisal edge position of the restoration. Special effects ceramic materials were layered (Fig C4-15) prior to final firing and glazing to establish proper surface luster (Fig C4-16); note the translucency of the synthetic ceramic material (HeraCeram [Heraeus-Kulzer-Jelenko, Armonk, NY]), as evidenced by the visibility of the prepared die through the restoration. The restoration was polished to achieve the final luster. After divestment, the veneer was fitted to the solid cast to establish proper proximal contacts and soft tissue emergence profile (Fig C4-17). Using the recommended shade protocol, a predictable and acceptable esthetic result was achieved with the fabrication of one restoration. The successful shade match was verified by ShadeScan before and after images (Fig C4-18), the ShadeVision virtual try-in (Fig C4-19), and the SpectroShade GBI map (Fig C4-20), as well as by the final clinical photographs (Figs C4-21 and C4-22).

Case 4: Single Anterior Ceramic Laminate Veneer

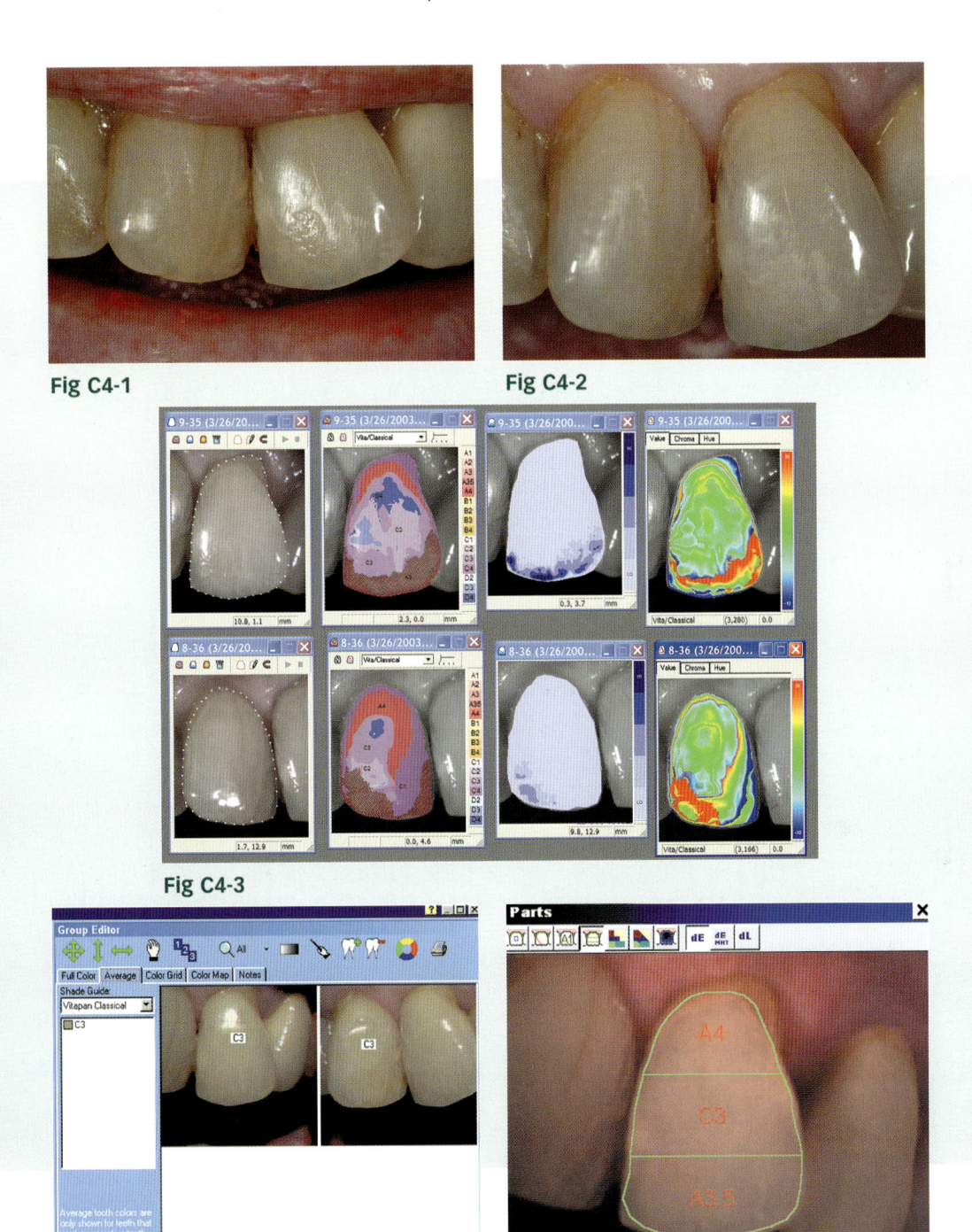

Fig C4-1

Fig C4-2

Fig C4-3

Fig C4-4

Fig C4-5

129

Appendix: Clinical Cases

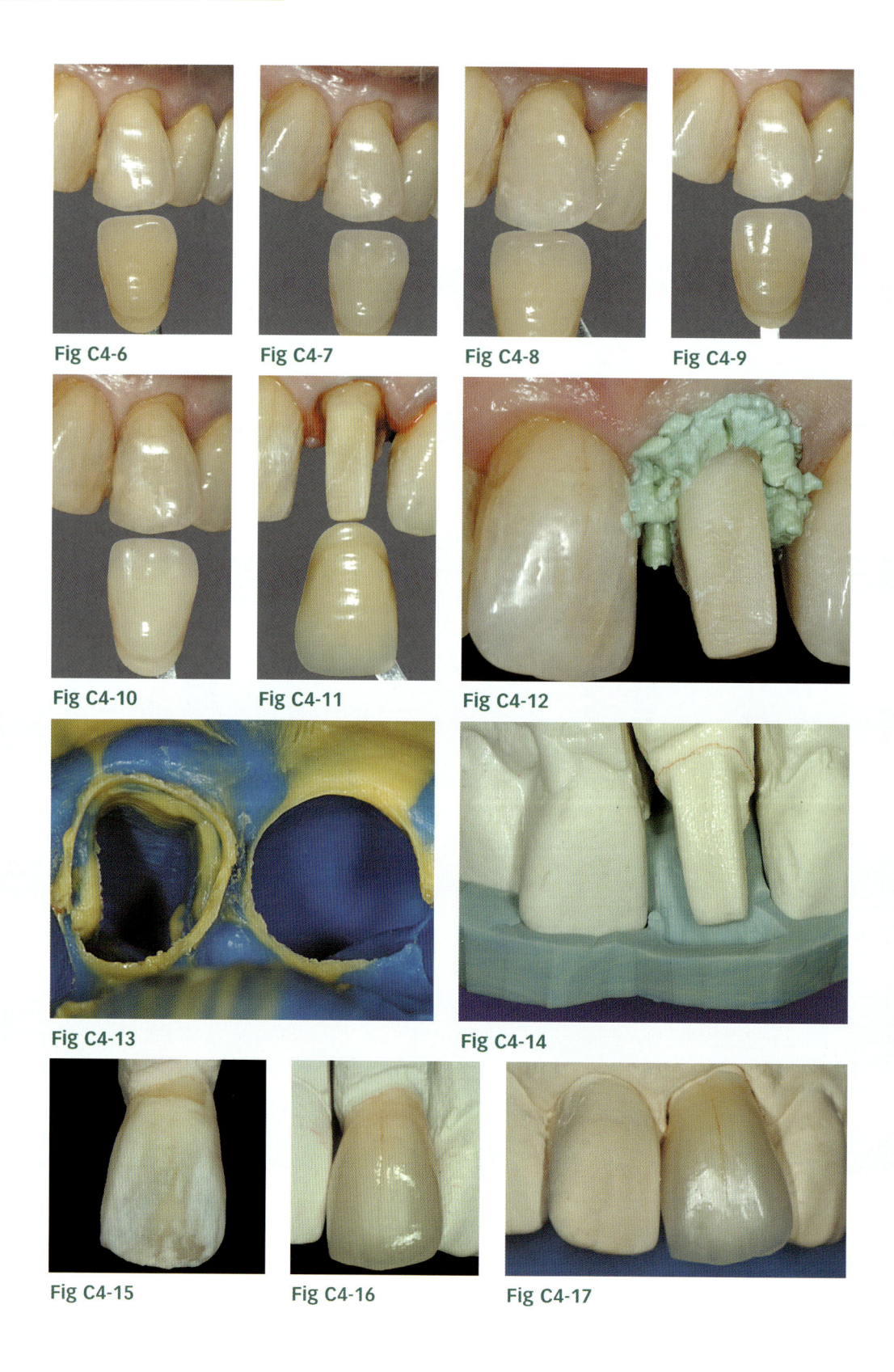

Fig C4-6

Fig C4-7

Fig C4-8

Fig C4-9

Fig C4-10

Fig C4-11

Fig C4-12

Fig C4-13

Fig C4-14

Fig C4-15

Fig C4-16

Fig C4-17

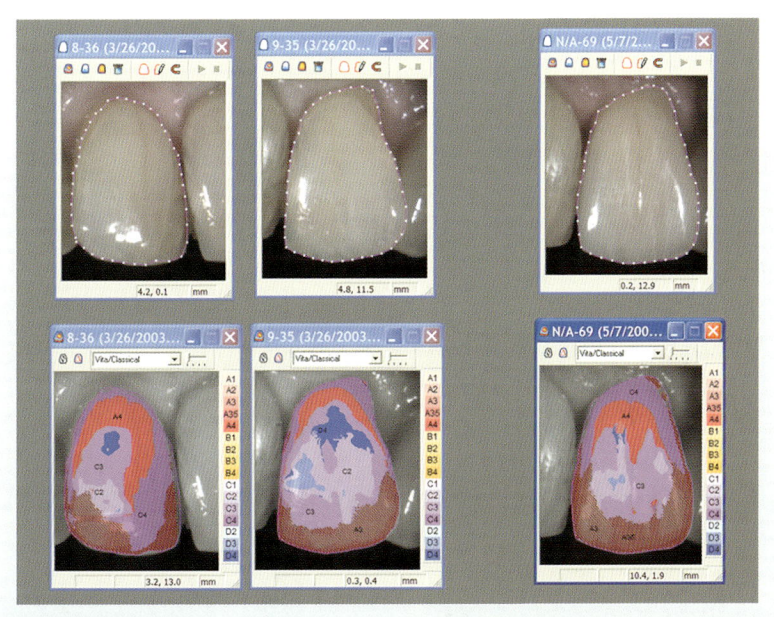

CASE 4: SINGLE ANTERIOR CERAMIC LAMINATE VENEER

Fig C4-18

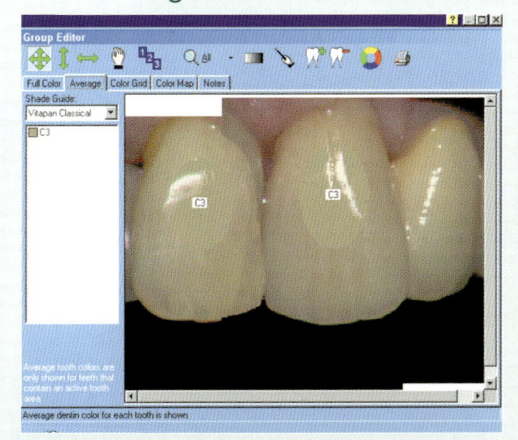

Fig C4-19

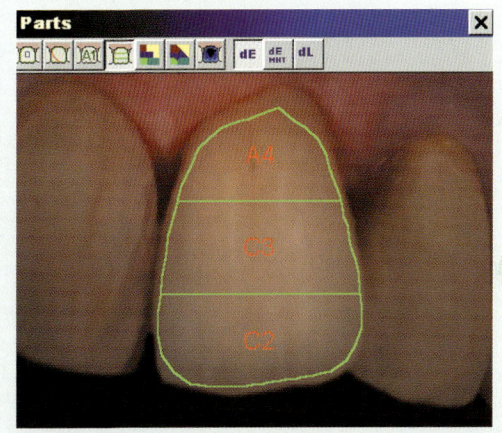

Fig C4-20

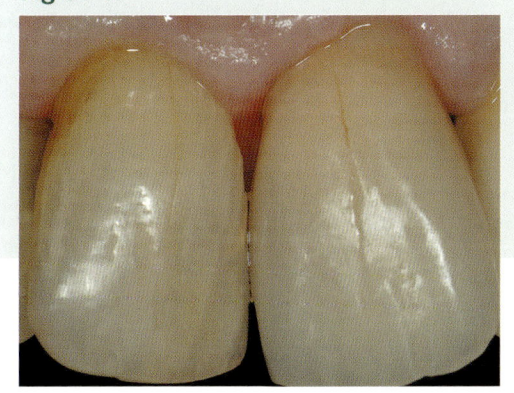

Fig C4-21

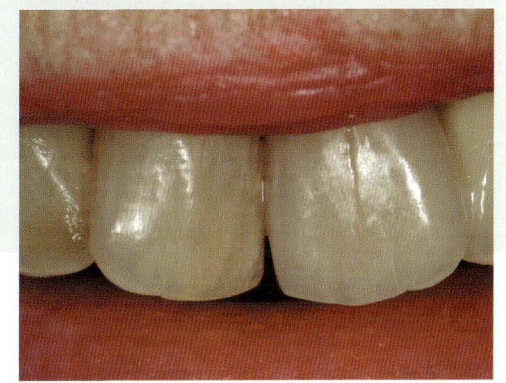

Fig C4-22

131

Appendix: Clinical Cases

Case 5: Two Anterior All-Ceramic Crowns

A 57-year-old woman presented with two maxillary lateral incisor crowns that did not match in shade and were causing gingival irritation due to poor emergence profile contours (Figs C5-1 to C5-3). Provisional restorations were made to allow the gingival tissues to heal. Close-up photographs of the central incisors were taken from different angles to communicate shade variations to the lab technician (Figs C5-4 and C5-5). A SpectroShade (MHT Optic Research, Niederhasli, Switzerland) GBI map was generated (Fig C5-6), based upon which reference photographs of shade tabs were taken (Figs C5-7 to C5-12). A reference photograph with the extreme shade tabs was also captured to assess value and chroma (Fig C5-13). The all-ceramic crowns (HeraCeram [Heraeus-Kulzer-Jelenko, Armonk, NY]) were fabricated in the lab, and the shade was visually verified. The proper embrasure and emergence profiles of the restorations were confirmed on the solid cast (Figs C5-14 to C5-17). Once the restorations were placed, the successful shade match was confirmed by the SpectroShade GBI maps (Figs C5-18 and C5-19) and clinical photographs (Figs C5-20 to C5-22).

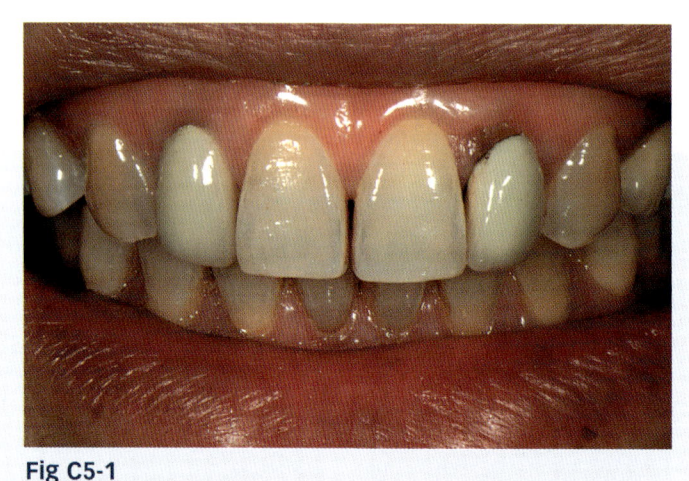

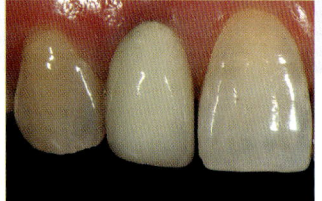

Fig C5-1

Fig C5-2

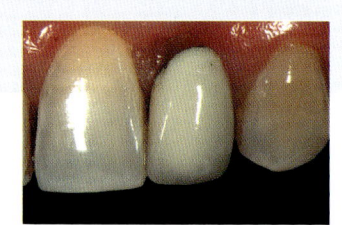

Fig C5-3

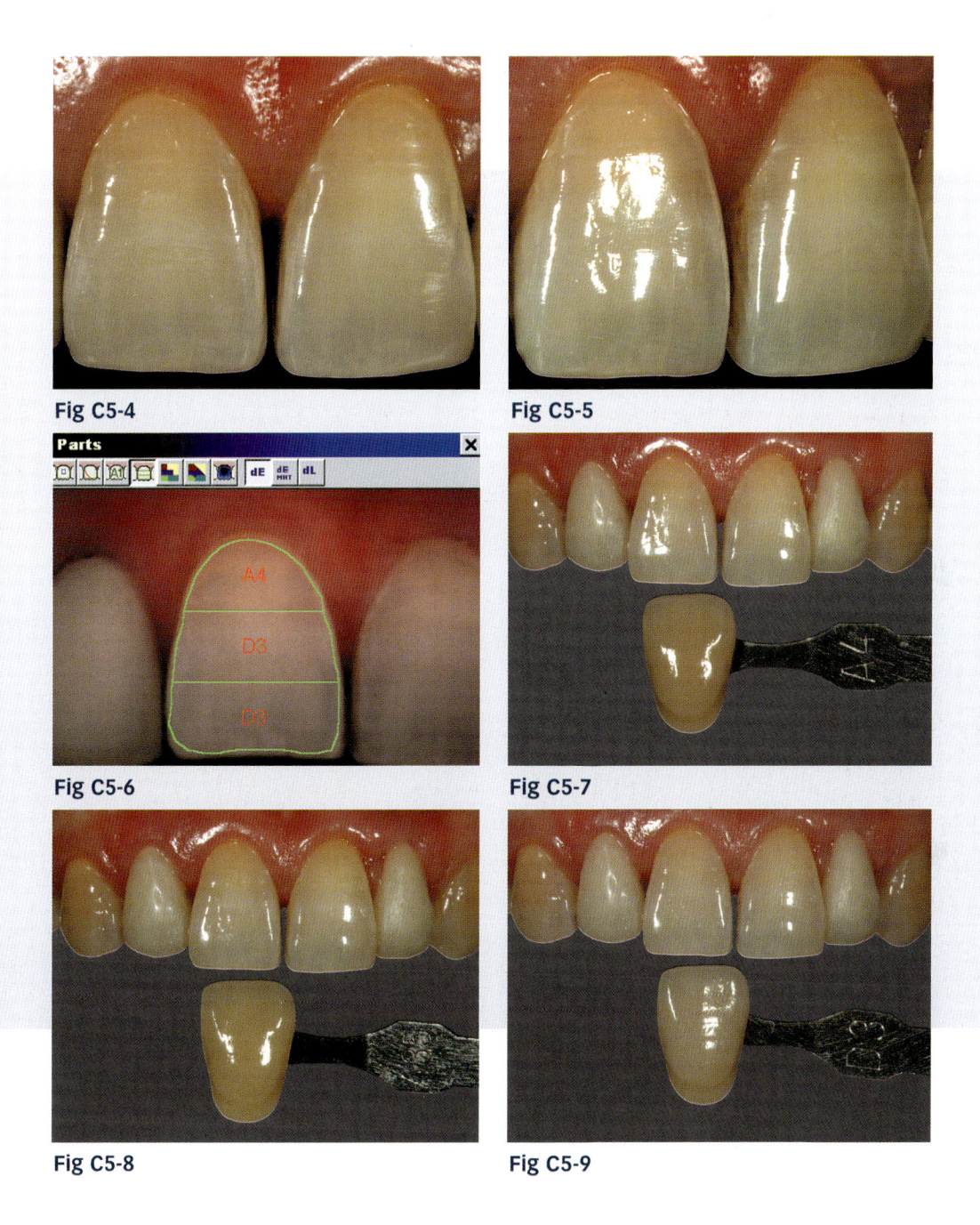

Case 5: Two Anterior All-Ceramic Crowns

Fig C5-4

Fig C5-5

Fig C5-6

Fig C5-7

Fig C5-8

Fig C5-9

133

Appendix: Clinical Cases

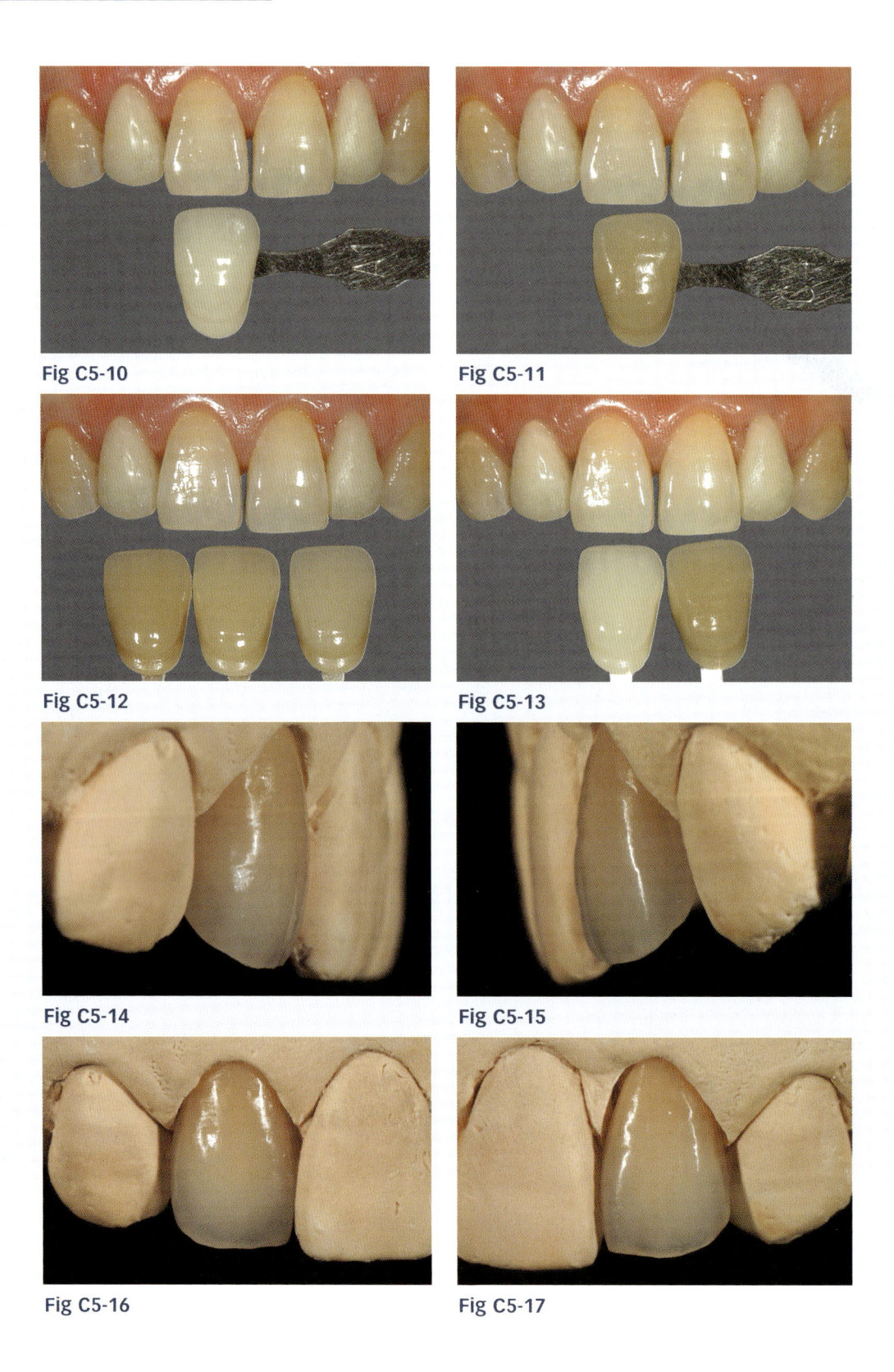

Fig C5-10

Fig C5-11

Fig C5-12

Fig C5-13

Fig C5-14

Fig C5-15

Fig C5-16

Fig C5-17

134

Case 5: Two Anterior All-Ceramic Crowns

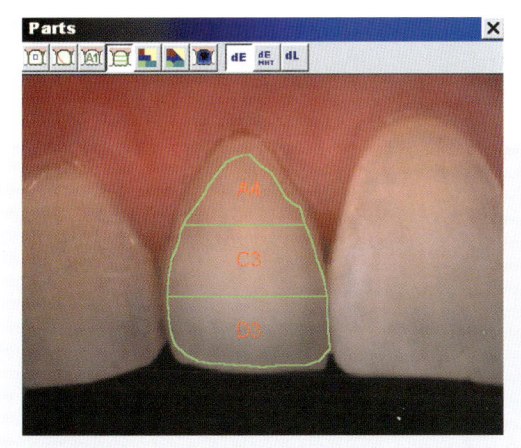

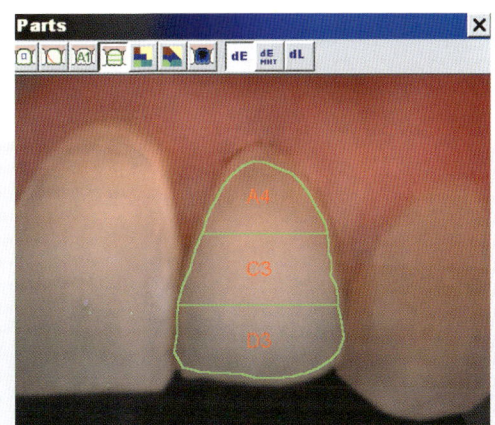

Fig C5-18

Fig C5-19

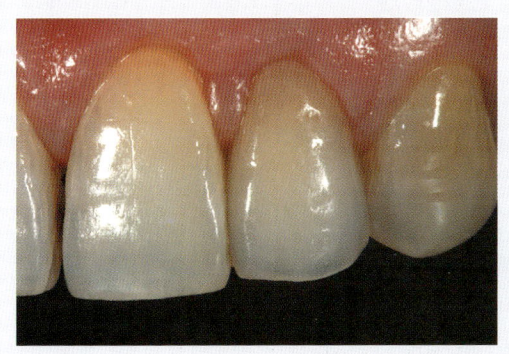

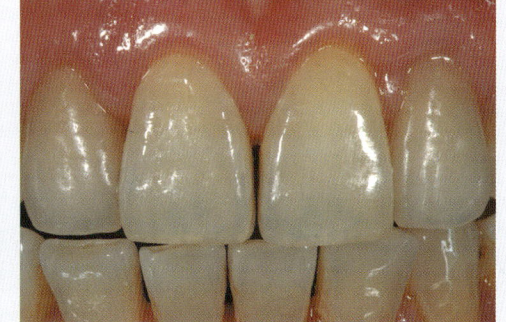

Fig C5-20

Fig C5-21

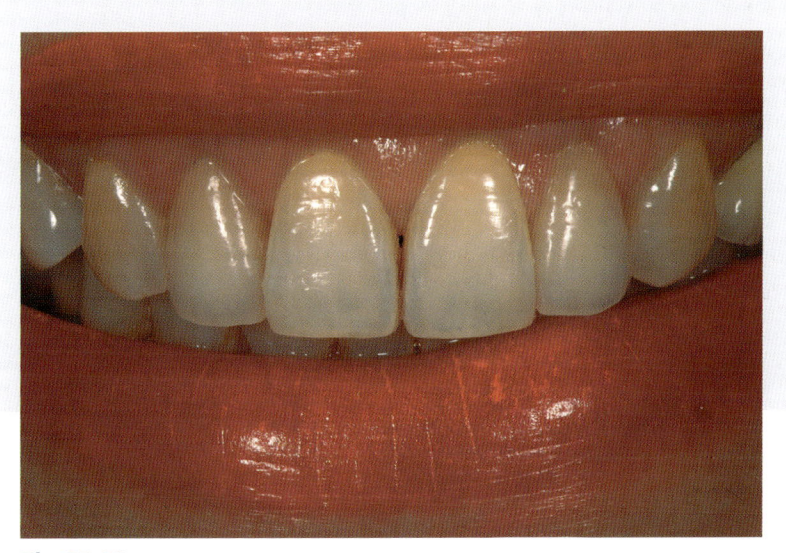

Fig C5-22

Appendix: Clinical Cases

Case 6: Two Anterior All-Ceramic Crowns with One Anterior Metal-Ceramic Crown

A 36-year-old man recently had received full-coverage crowns on his maxillary central incisors and left lateral incisor with an extremely dissatisfactory result (Figs C6-1 and C6-2). Root canal therapy had been performed on both lateral incisors, with the left receiving an alloy post-core foundation restoration, which discolored the remaining tooth structure due to oxidation of the alloy post (Fig C6-3). The right central incisor preparation was slightly more discolored than the left central incisor because of precipitation of ferric sulfide salts into the dentinal tubules following root canal therapy (see Fig C6-3).

Provisional restorations were made to restore proper form, proportion, and incisal length and as a blueprint for the definitive restorations (Fig C6-4). ShadeScan (Cynovad, Montreal, Canada) (Fig C6-5), ShadeVision (X-Rite, Grandville, MI) (Fig C6-6), and SpectroShade (MHT Optic Research, Niederhasli, Switzerland) (Figs C6-7 to C6-9) were used to determine the shade of the natural dentition. Shade communication was performed using reference photographs with the shade tabs suggested by the technology-based shade analysis (Figs C6-10 to C6-13), as well as extreme shade tabs for value and chroma assessment (Figs C6-14 and C6-15). All-ceramic refractory crowns were selected for the central incisors, and an alloy-reinforced crown was selected for the left lateral incisor to mask the discolored preparation and root (Fig C6-16). The restorations were baked and shaped, and proper surface texture and luster were created (Fig C6-17). The restorations were evaluated for correct depth of incisal effects, translucency, and light transmission (eg, blue opalescence shown in Fig C6-18). The ShadeVision virtual try-in visually verified accurate shade reproduction (Fig C6-19). The SpectroShade compared synchronized images to establish an aggregate ΔE value of less than 2.0, which confirmed a very close match (Fig C6-20), as seen in the clinical photographs of the final restorations (Figs C6-21 and C6-22). The use of different restorative materials was integral to achieving the desired esthetic result.

Case 6: Anterior All-Ceramic Crowns with Anterior Metal-Ceramic Crown

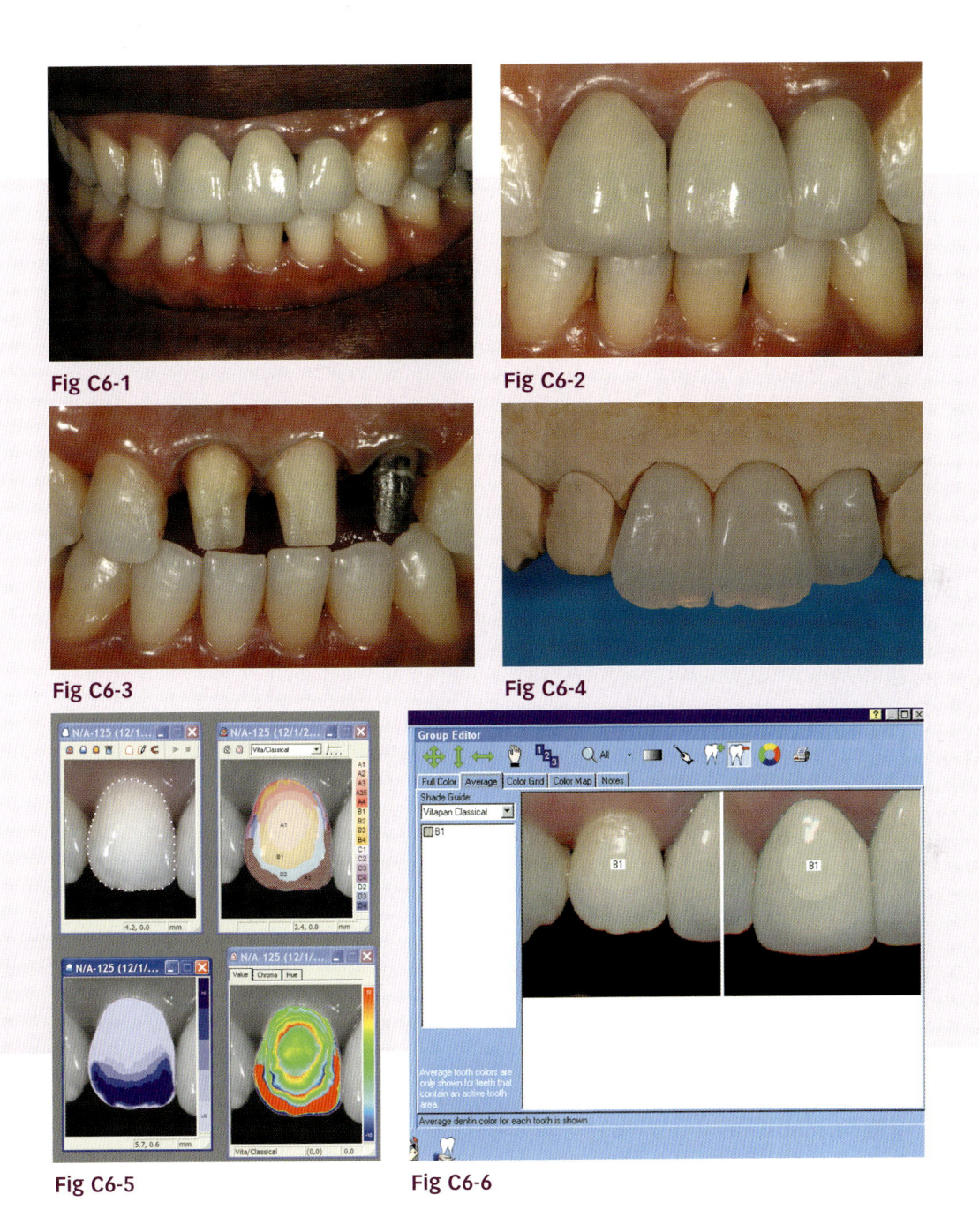

Fig C6-1

Fig C6-2

Fig C6-3

Fig C6-4

Fig C6-5

Fig C6-6

137

APPENDIX: CLINICAL CASES

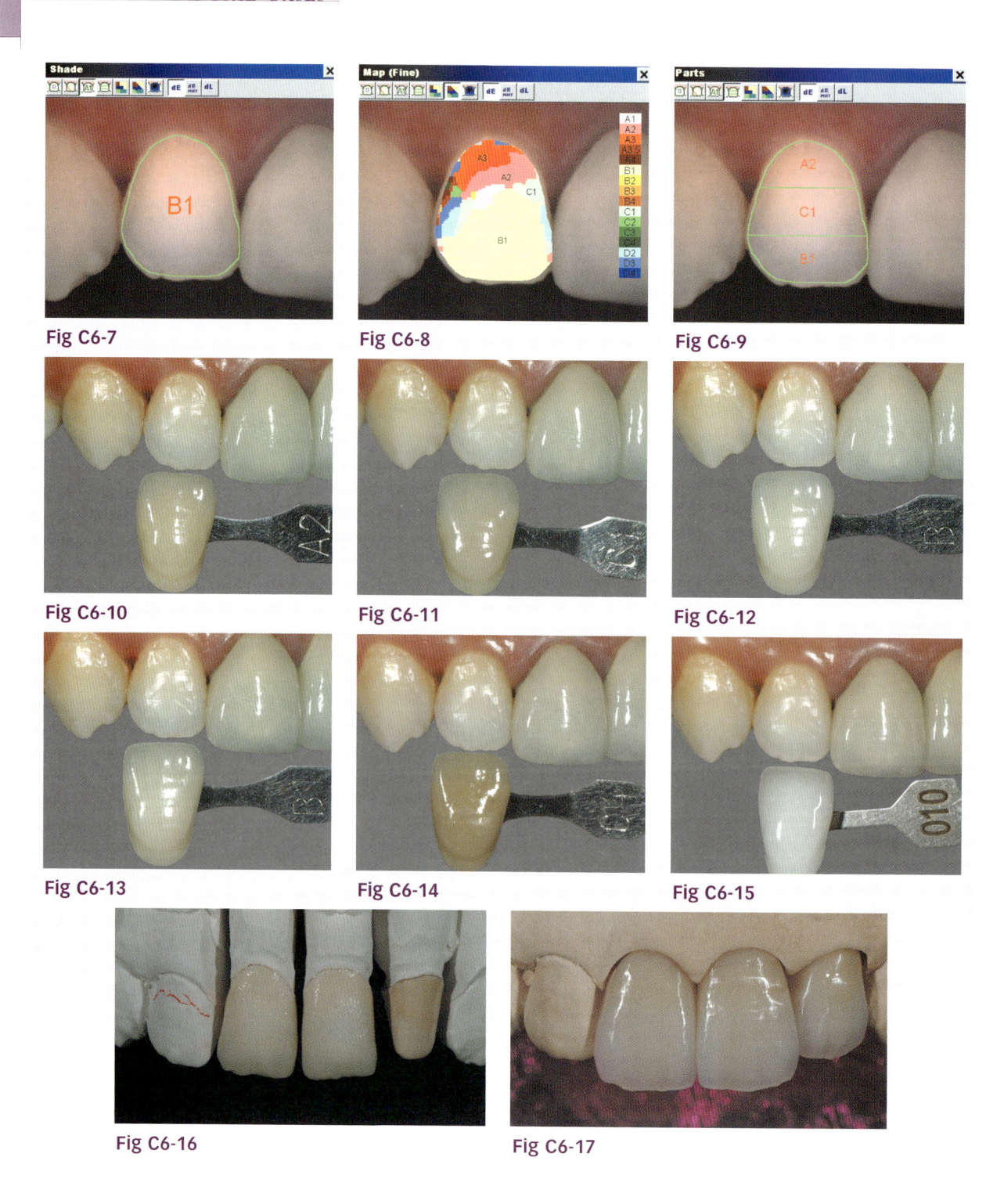

Fig C6-7

Fig C6-8

Fig C6-9

Fig C6-10

Fig C6-11

Fig C6-12

Fig C6-13

Fig C6-14

Fig C6-15

Fig C6-16

Fig C6-17

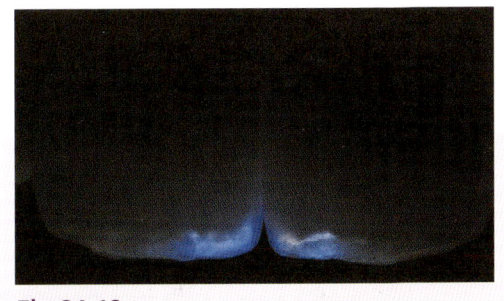

Case 6: Anterior All-Ceramic Crowns with Anterior Metal-Ceramic Crown

Fig C6-18

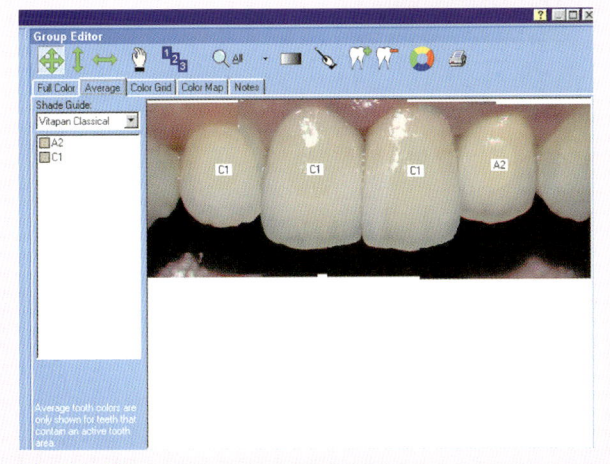

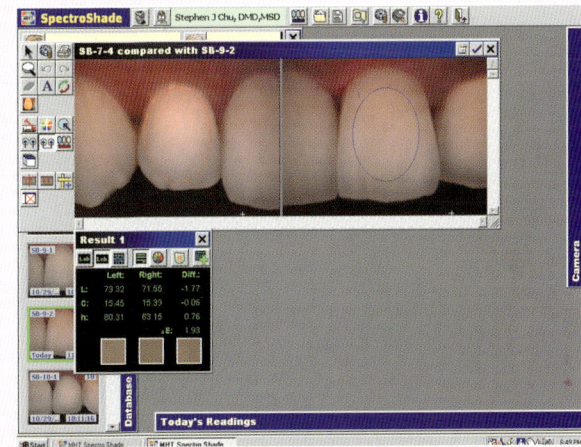

Fig C6-19

Fig C6-20

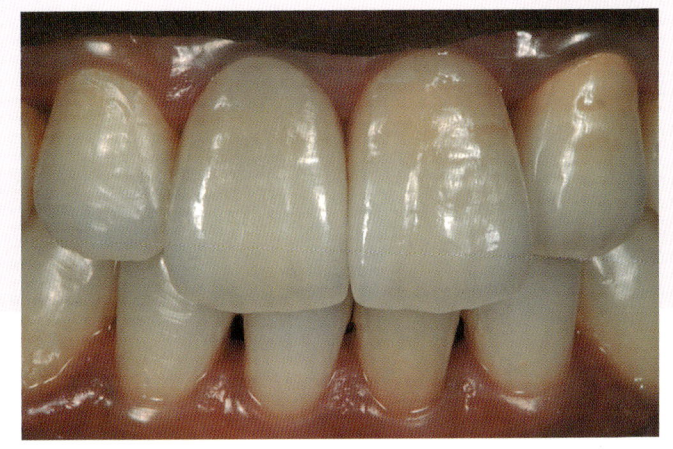

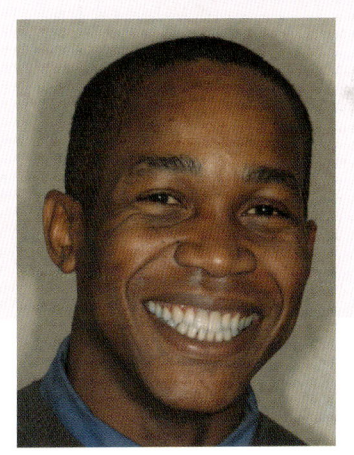

Fig C6-21

Fig C6-22

139

Appendix: Clinical Cases

Case 7: Four Anterior Ceramic Laminate Veneers

A 25-year-old woman presented with a chief complaint of being dissatisfied with the esthetic appearance of four anterior (pressable leucite-reinforced) ceramic veneers (Empress [Ivoclar-Vivadent, Amherst, NY]), which had been made for her maxillary lateral and central incisors 2 years prior (Fig C7-1). Clinical examination revealed discrepancies in the color, value, and proportion of the veneers (Fig C7-2). Moreover, the teeth had a square shape, as confirmed by measurement with a periodontal probe, which indicated a 100% length-to-width ratio (Figs C7-3 and C7-4). Radiographic evaluation revealed peg-shaped lateral incisors (Figs C7-5 and C7-6), and it was determined that space could be gained at the expense of the distal aspects of the central incisors, which would decrease their width and create proper proportion for the four incisors.

A composite mock-up was performed (Fig C7-7) and the teeth prepared to receive new all-ceramic restorations (Fig C7-8). A paste deflection tissue management system (Fig C7-9) was used prior to final impression making (Fig C7-10). The ShadeVision (X-Rite, Grandville, MI) system was used for shade analysis, and Vitapan (Vita, Bad Sackingen, Germany) shade B1 was reported (Figs C7-11 and C7-12). A diagnostic waxup was made to control final tooth contours and dimensions pretreatment (Fig C7-13) and posttreatment (Fig C7-14). The ceramic three-quarter laminate veneers were baked on a refractory cast employing the incisal matrix technique (Figs C7-15 and C7-16). The veneers were then fitted to the solid cast to define contact areas, gingival embrasures, and emergence profiles (Fig C7-17). A virtual try-in was performed, and shade was visually assessed and approved prior to adhesive cementation (Fig C7-18). The final ShadeVision report confirmed that the Vitapan B1 shade was successfully matched (Fig C7-19), and the clinical presentation confirmed the successful shade match with the surrounding dentition, as well as the improvement in the tooth proportions (Figs C7-20 and C7-21).

Case 7: Four Anterior Ceramic Laminate Veneers

Fig C7-1

Fig C7-2

Fig C7-3

Fig C7-4

Fig C7-5

Fig C7-6

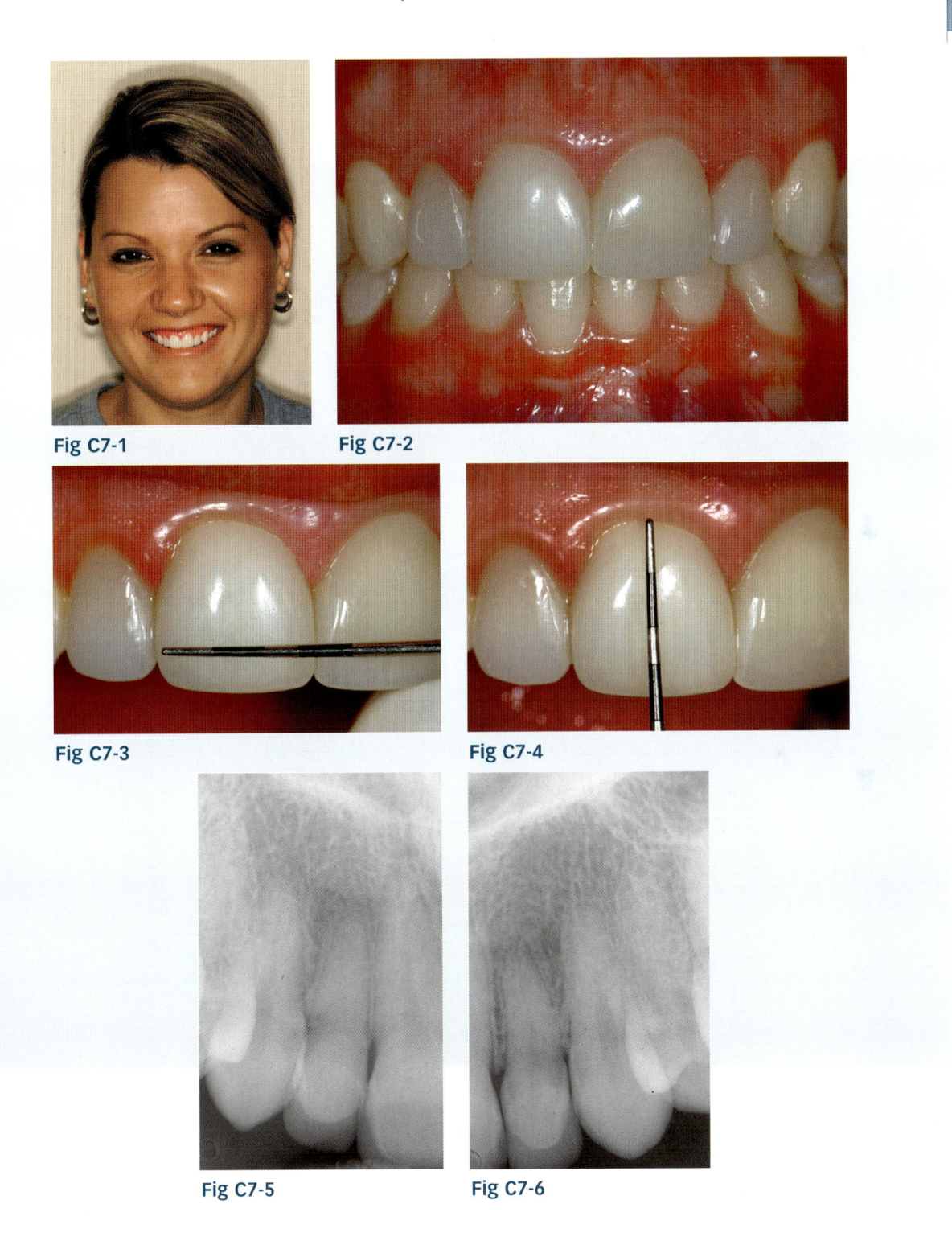

141

Appendix: Clinical Cases

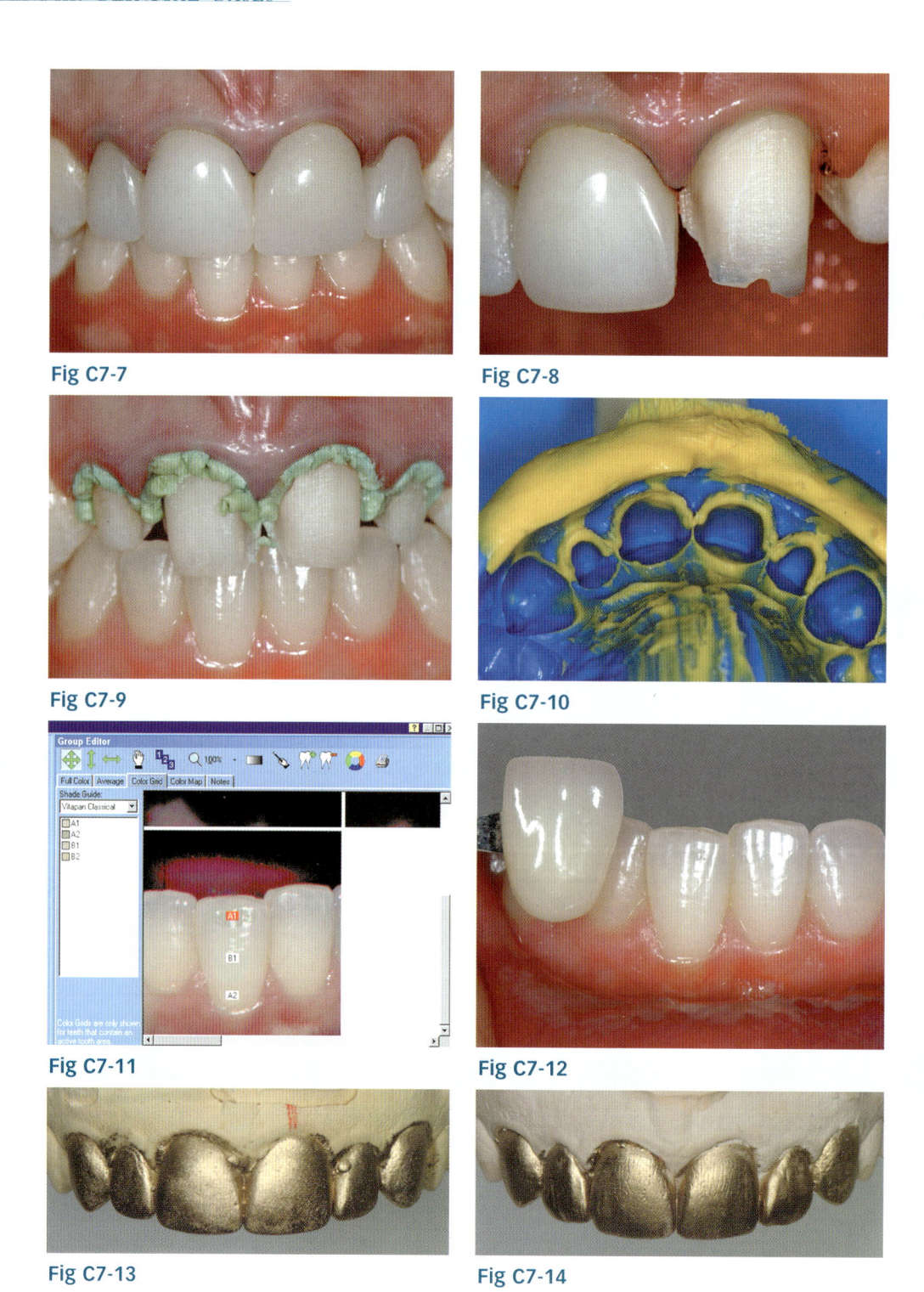

Fig C7-7

Fig C7-8

Fig C7-9

Fig C7-10

Fig C7-11

Fig C7-12

Fig C7-13

Fig C7-14

Case 7: Four Anterior Ceramic Laminate Veneers

Fig C7-15

Fig C7-16

Fig C7-17

Fig C7-18

Fig C7-19

Fig C7-20

Fig C7-21

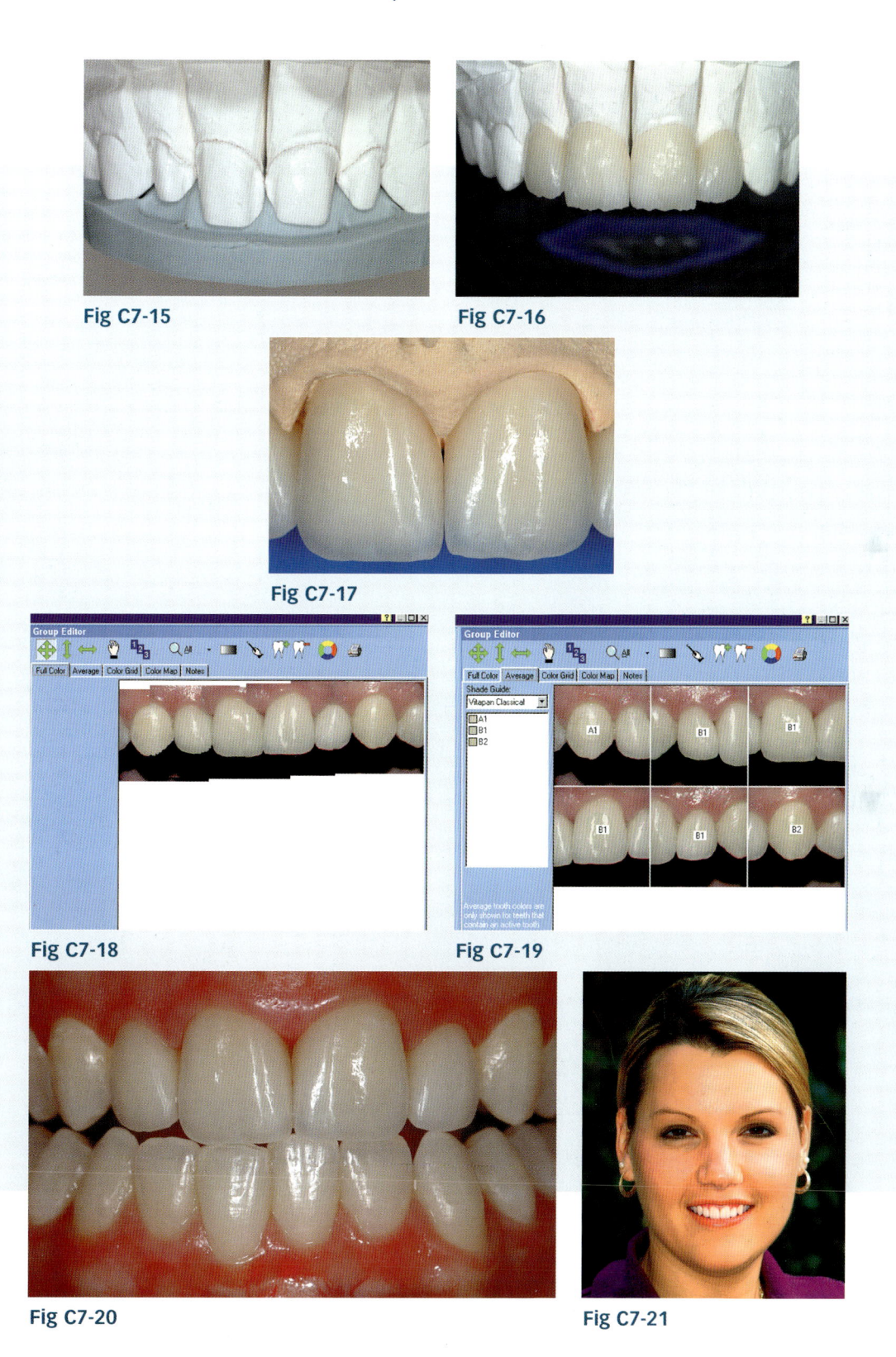

143

APPENDIX: CLINICAL CASES

Case 8: Single Posterior All-Ceramic Crown

A maxillary left premolar with an existing large mesio-occlusodistal direct composite restoration was prepared for an all-ceramic full-coverage restoration because of extensive recurrent proximal and cervical caries (Figs C8-1 to C8-3). Shade analysis was performed using the ShadeScan (Cynovad, Montreal, Canada) system, and a Vitapan (Vita, Bad Sackingen, Germany) B1/A1 shade was determined (Fig C8-4). Technology-based shade matching alone was used in this case, which is often adequate when only the posterior teeth are involved. The ceramic system and the appropriate ceramic powders were selected during shade determination. A refractory cast technique was used to fabricate the crown (Figs C8-5 to C8-15). The crown was placed using a resin composite cement system (Lute-it [Pentron, Wallingford, CT]), and an esthetic shade match was achieved (Figs C8-16 to C8-18).

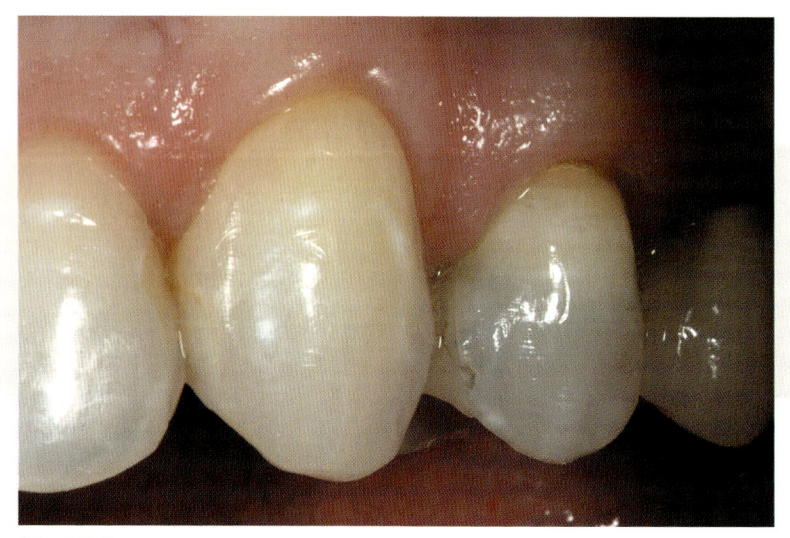

Fig C8-1

CASE 8: SINGLE POSTERIOR ALL-CERAMIC CROWN

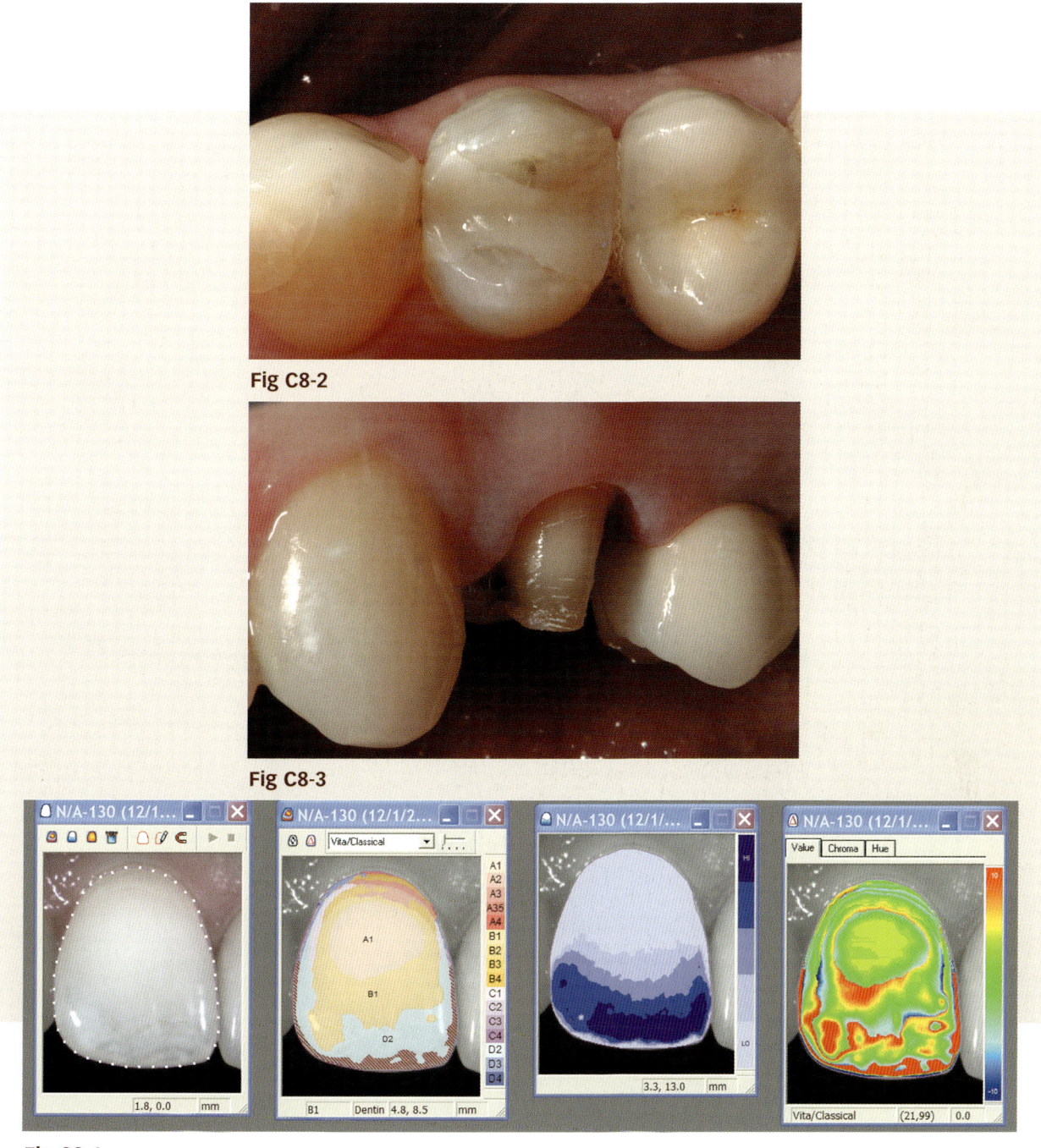

Fig C8-2

Fig C8-3

Fig C8-4

145

Appendix: Clinical Cases

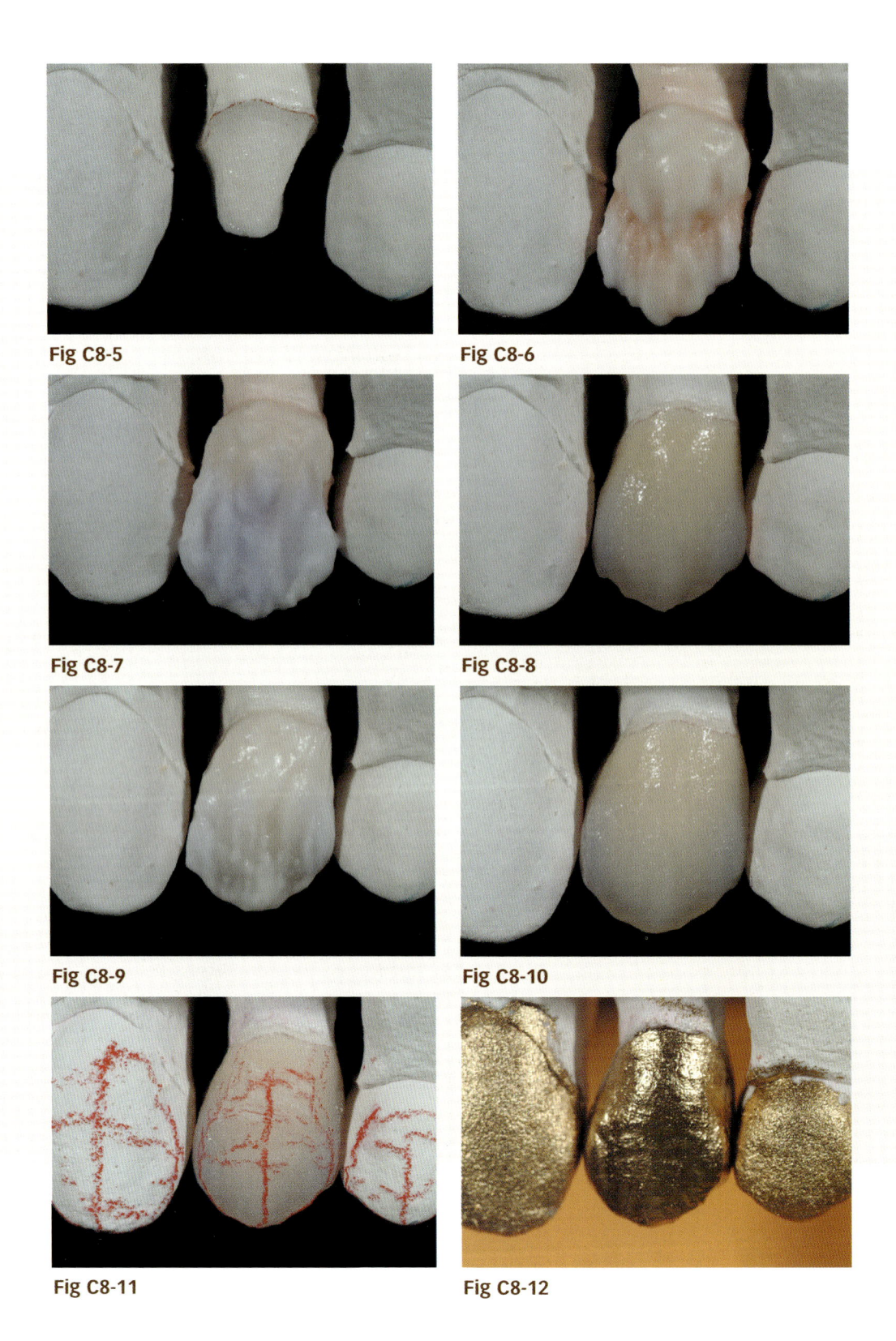

Fig C8-5

Fig C8-6

Fig C8-7

Fig C8-8

Fig C8-9

Fig C8-10

Fig C8-11

Fig C8-12

CASE 8: SINGLE POSTERIOR ALL-CERAMIC CROWN

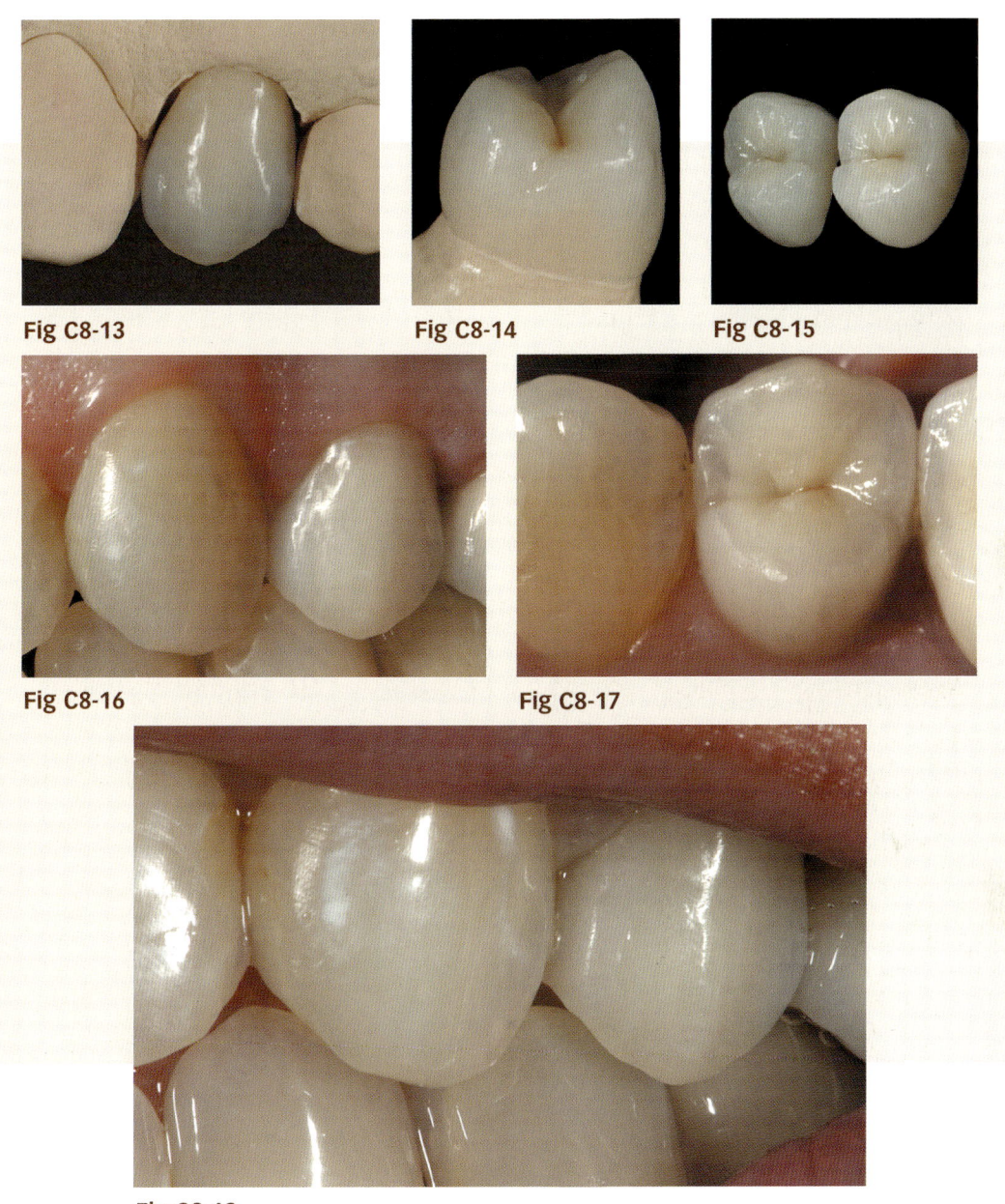

Fig C8-13

Fig C8-14

Fig C8-15

Fig C8-16

Fig C8-17

Fig C8-18

APPENDIX: CLINICAL CASES

Case 9: Ten Ceramic Laminate Veneers to Match Bleached Teeth

A 50-year-old woman presented with existing composite veneer facings, large interproximal restorations, recurrent caries, and discoloration localized to the maxillary dentition. Dentofacial analysis photographs revealed incorrect tooth proportions and excessive gingival display in the posterior dentition (Figs C9-1 and C9-2). Prior to esthetic restorative treatment, the mandibular dentition was whitened using a professional take-home vital bleaching system (Colgate Platinum [Colgate-Palmolive, New York, NY]). A composite mock-up was done to re-establish proper tooth proportions (Fig C9-3), and controlled-depth tooth reduction was performed (Fig C9-4). Subsequently, existing interproximal restorations and recurrent decay were removed (Fig C9-5). The ShadeVision (X-Rite, Grandville, MI) system was used for shade analysis, and a Vitapan (Vita, Bad Sackingen, Germany) D2 gingival shade and a B1 bleached body and incisal shade were selected (Fig C9-6). These shades were confirmed visually using conventional shade tabs (Figs C9-7 to C9-9). A refractory cast technique was used to fabricate the ceramic veneer restorations (Fig C9-10), and many internal cracks and craze lines were layered into the ceramic buildup to match the characterization of the natural dentition (Fig C9-11). The final ShadeVision report verified a precise clinical and colorimetric shade match to the bleached natural mandibular dentition (Fig C9-12), which is confirmed by clinical photographs (Figs C9-13 and C9-14).

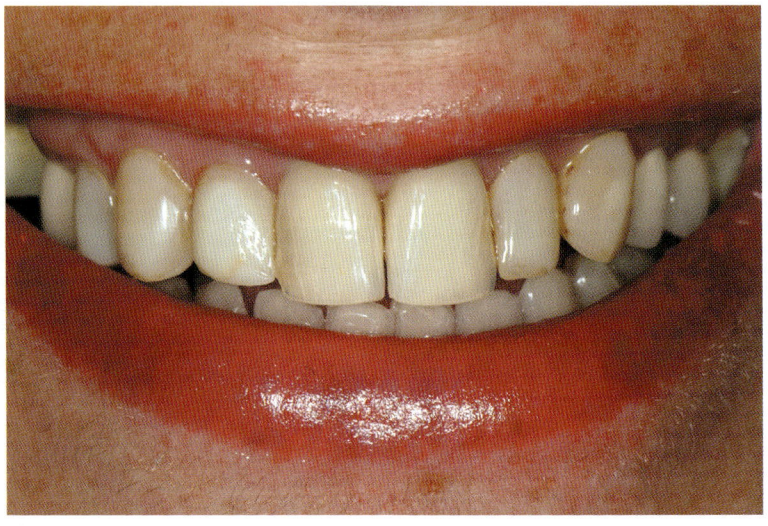

Fig C9-1

Case 9: Ten Ceramic Laminate Veneers to Match Bleached Teeth

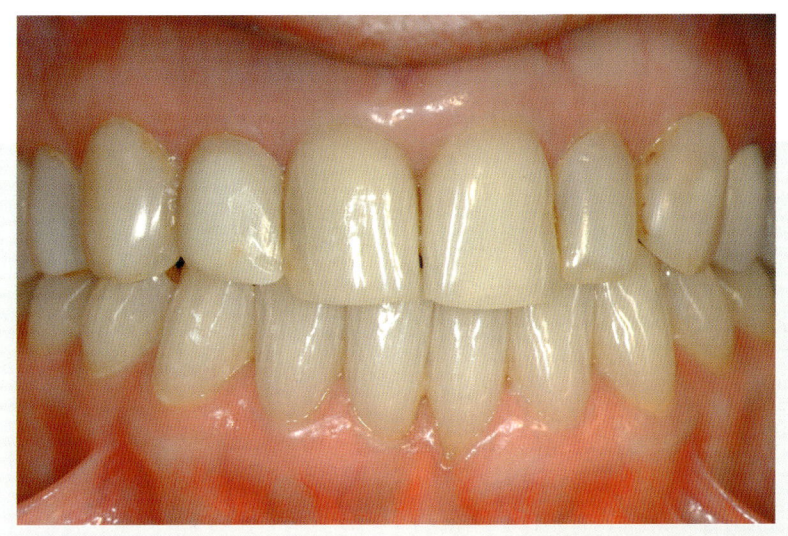

Fig C9-2

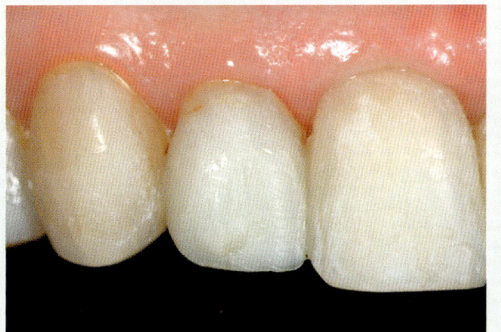

Fig C9-3

Fig C9-4

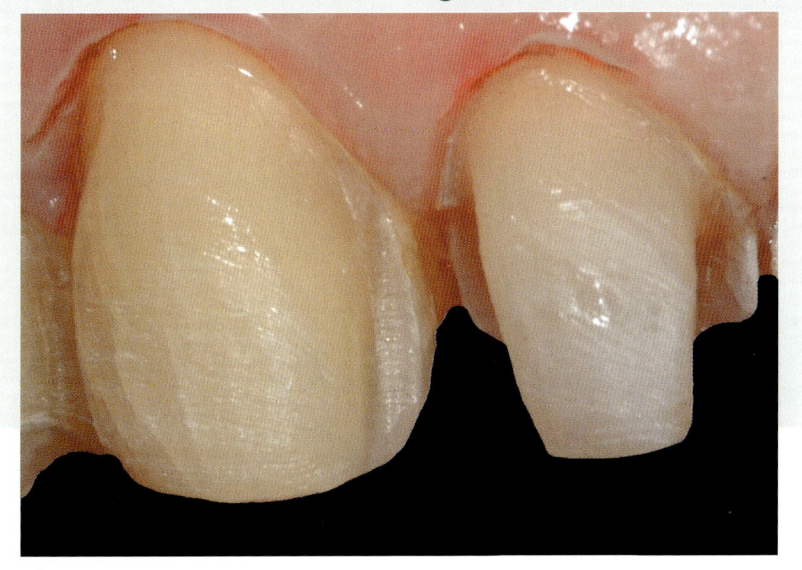

Fig C9-5

149

Appendix: Clinical Cases

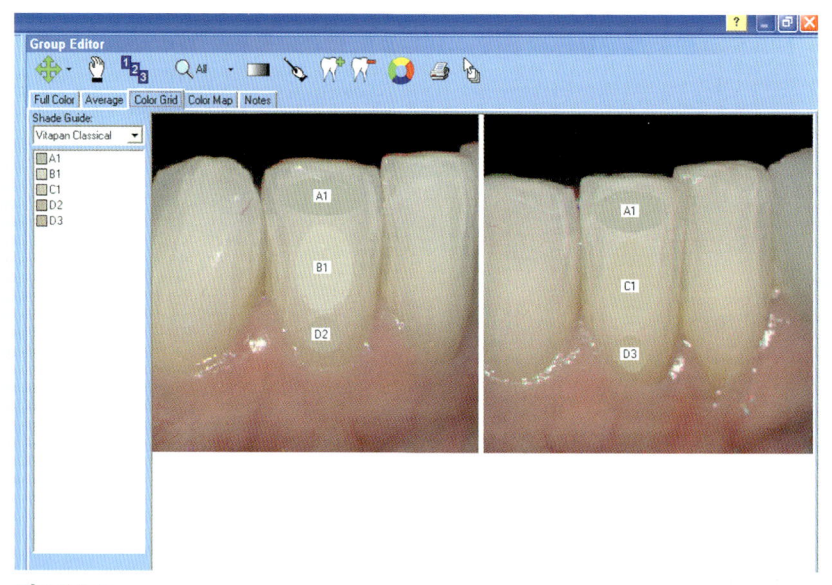

Fig C9-6

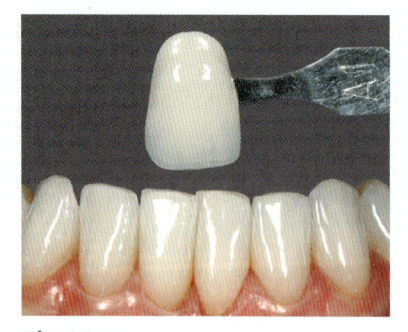

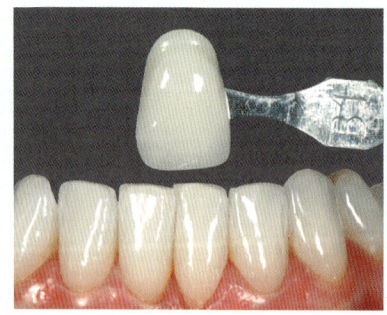

Fig C9-7

Fig C9-8

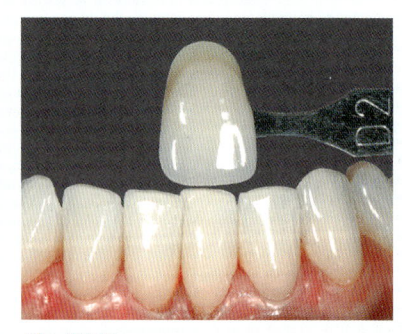

Fig C9-9

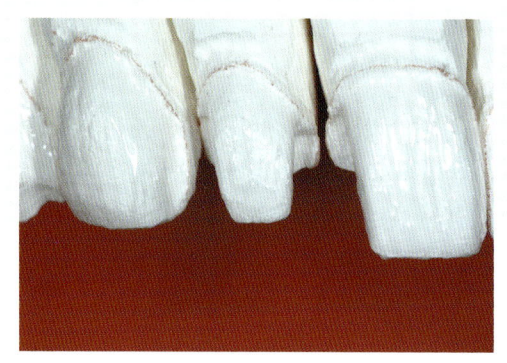

Fig C9-10

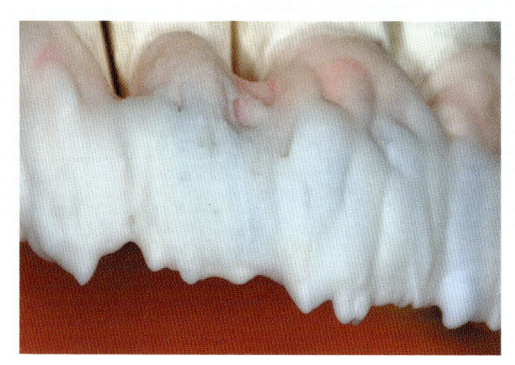

Fig C9-11

150

Case 9: Ten Ceramic Laminate Veneers to Match Bleached Teeth

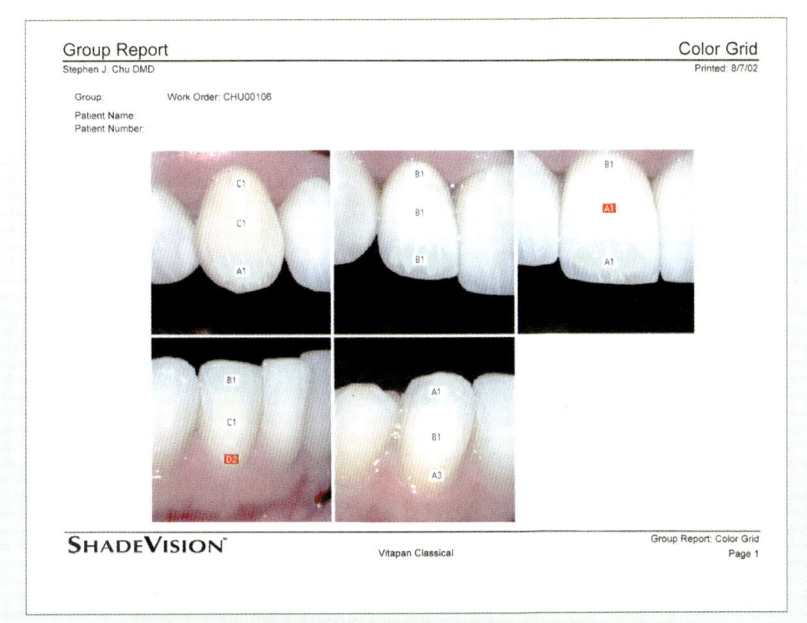

Fig C9-12

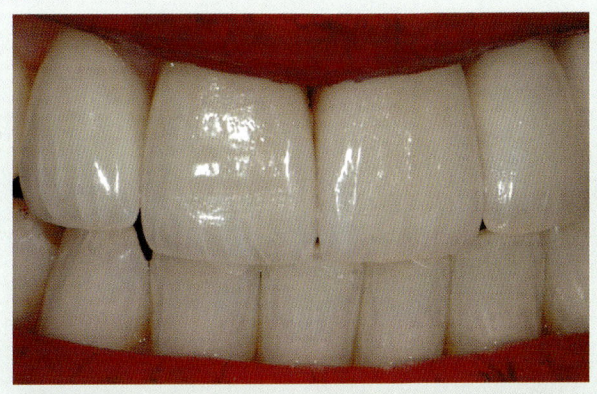

Fig C9-13

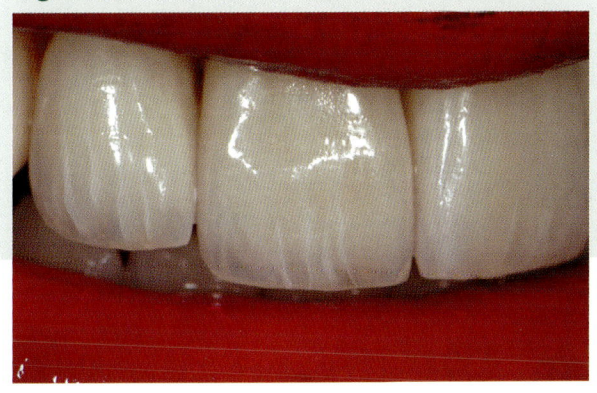

Fig C9-14

Appendix: Clinical Cases

Case 10: Two Anterior Direct Composite Restorations

A 30-year-old woman presented with generalized cervical caries as a consequence of poor diet and nonfluoridation of the drinking water system during growth and development (Figs C10-1 to C10-3).

The SpectroShade (MHT Optic Research, Niederhasli, Switzerland) system was used for shade analysis (Fig C10-4), and a Vitapan (Vita, Bad Sackingen, Germany) D3 shade was selected. Conventional shade tabs were used to confirm the shade (Fig C10-5). A direct composite adhesive system (Gradia [GC America, Chicago, IL]) was used to restore the cervical lesions following caries removal (Figs C10-6 to C10-11). The shade was verified using the SpectroShade device after finishing (Fig C10-12). Technology-based shade analysis facilitated the esthetic outcome and clinical success of these direct composite restorations (Figs C10-13 and C10-14).

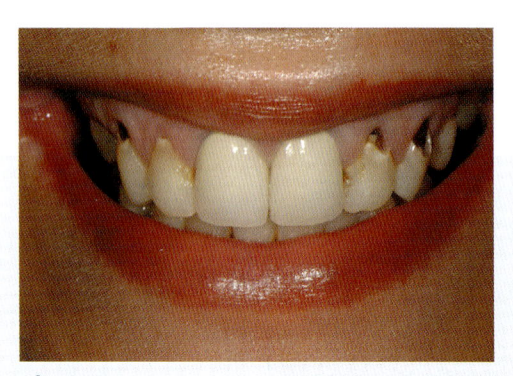

Fig C10-1

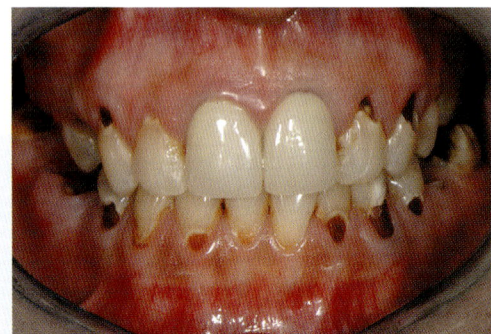

Fig C10-2

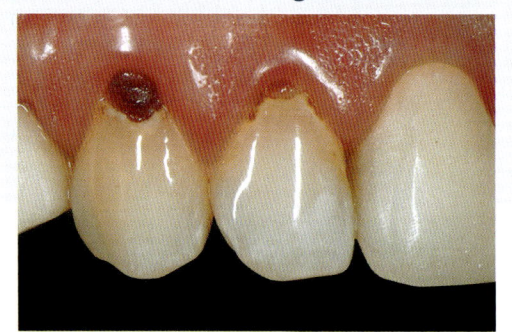

Fig C10-3

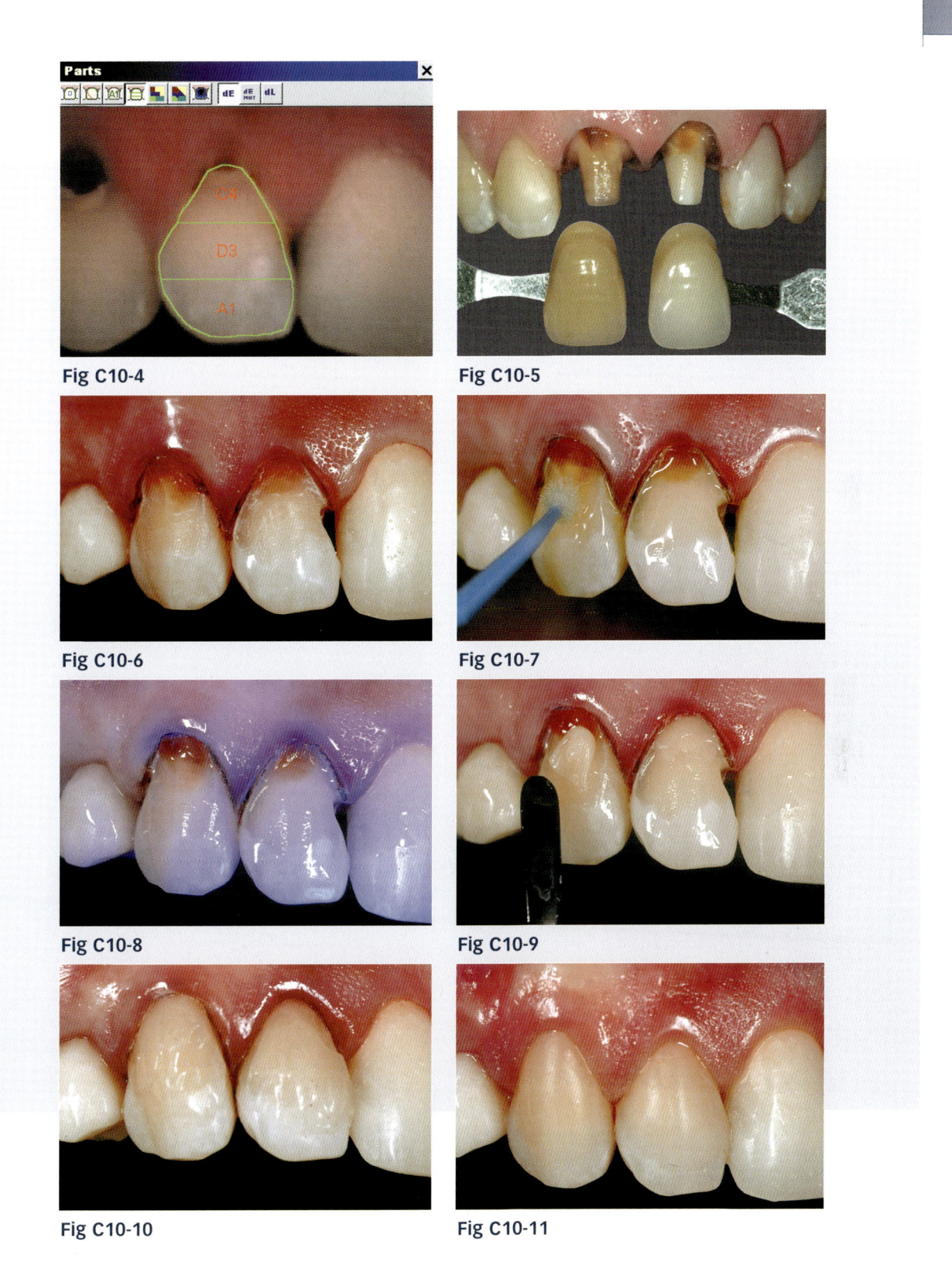

CASE 10: TWO ANTERIOR DIRECT COMPOSITE RESTORATIONS

Fig C10-4

Fig C10-5

Fig C10-6

Fig C10-7

Fig C10-8

Fig C10-9

Fig C10-10

Fig C10-11

153

Appendix: Clinical Cases

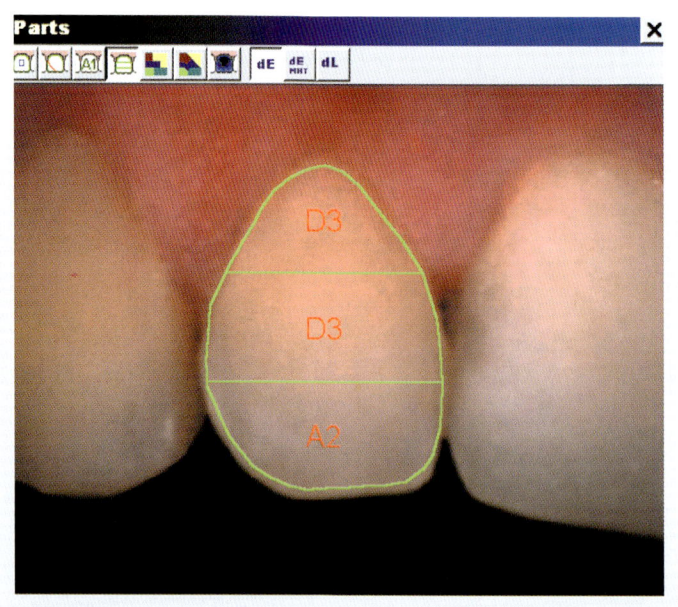

Fig C10-12

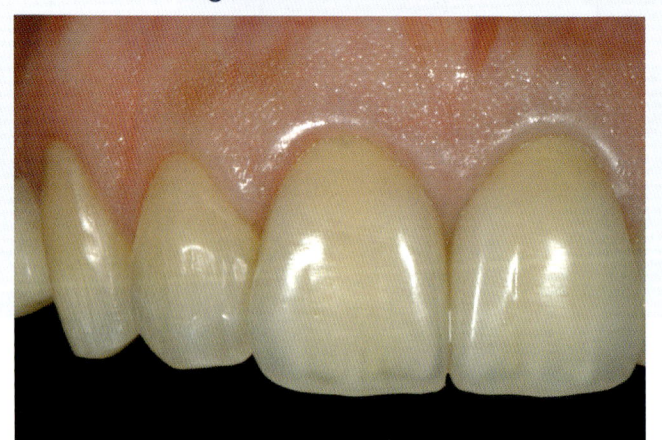

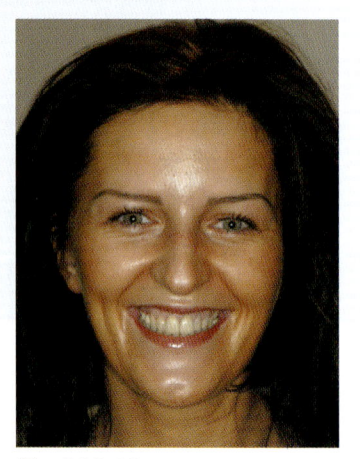

Fig C10-13

Fig C10-14

Index

Page numbers followed by "f" denote figures and "t" denote tables

A

Absorption of light, 4–7
Additive primary colors, 10
Adolescents, 90, 90f
Aging
 color matching affected by, 39
 tooth structure changes, 90, 90f–91f
"Alfred E. Newman" expectations, 54, 55f
All-ceramic crowns
 In-Ceram, 122–123
 Procera, 118–121
 single anterior, 118–123
 single posterior, 144–147
 two anterior, 132–139
Analysis
 for conventional shade matching, 52–55, 53f–55f
 for recommended shade-matching protocol, 104, 104f–105f
 for technological shade matching, 87–88
Anterior ceramic laminate veneers
 four, 140–143
 single, 128–131
Anterior direct composite restorations, 152–154
Antioxidants, 40
Areal contrast, 31t, 36, 36f

B

Binocular difference, 42, 42f
Bleached teeth
 anterior ceramic laminate veneers matched to, 148–151
 color matching of, 53
 description of, 43–44, 44f, 47–48
Blue, 4t, 13
Bluish translucency, 16f
Brightness, 8

C

Case studies
 all-ceramic crowns
  In-Ceram, 122–123
  Procera, 118–121
  single anterior, 118–123
  two anterior, 132–139
 anterior ceramic laminate veneers
  bleached teeth matched to, 148–151
  four, 140–143
  single, 128–131
 direct composite restorations, 152–154
 implant-supported metal-ceramic crown, 124–127
Cast, 67f
Ceramic laminate veneers, anterior
 four, 140–143
 single, 128–131
Ceramics
 fracture toughness of, 44t
 translucency of, 44t

Chroma
 of bleached teeth, 52, 53f
 dentinal, 72, 72f
 description of, 15–16
 determination of, 61
Chroma contrast, 31t, 35, 35f
Chromascop shade guide, 60
Classic layering concept, 70, 71f
Clinician–laboratory communication, 56f, 56–57, 89
CMY(K) color model, 10–12
Color(s)
 aging effects on, 91
 of bleached teeth, 43–44, 44f
 brightness of, 8
 complementary, 14, 14f
 description of, 2
 dimensions of, 14–16
 elements necessary for, 2
 physics of, 3–8
 pigment, 12–14, 13t
 primary. *See* Primary colors.
 secondary, 13, 13f
 types of, 3
 wavelengths of, 3, 4t
Color blindness, 38–39
Color matching. *See* Shade matching.
Color models
 CMY(K), 10–12
 RGB, 10
Color perception
 binocular difference in, 42, 42f
 emotions effect on, 40–41
 factors that affect, 2, 31–32

155

Index

fatigue effects on, 40
medications effect on, 41, 41t
physiology of, 8, 9f
processes involved in, 4–5, 8
realities of, 9t
Color reproduction
  CMY(K) color model, 10–12
  description of, 9
  RGB color model, 10
Color spectrum, 3
Color temperature, 57, 57f
Color temperature meter, 27
Color vision problem, 38–39
Color wheel, 14–15
Color-corrected lighting, 27, 28f
Colorimeters, 86–87
Commission Internationale de l'Eclairage (CIE), 21–22
Communication
  for conventional shade matching, 56f, 56–57
  for recommended shade-matching protocol, 106, 106f–107f
  for technological shade matching, 89
Complementary colors, 14, 14f
Complete-tooth measurement devices, 80–81
Cones, 3, 8, 8f, 39
Contrast
  areal, 31t, 36, 36f
  chroma, 31t, 35, 35f
  definition of, 30
  hue, 31t, 33–34, 34f
  simultaneous, 31–35
  spatial, 31t, 37, 37f
  successive, 31t, 37–38, 38f
  value, 31t, 32f–33f, 32–33
Conventional shade matching
  direct composites. See Direct composite restorations.
  protocol for, 62–63, 63f–69f
  shade guides, 59–61, 64f
  steps involved in analysis, 52–55

communication, 56f, 56–57
fabrication, 58f, 58–59
interpretation, 58
verification, 59, 59f
Crowns
  all-ceramic
    In-Ceram, 122–123
    Procera, 118–121
    single anterior, 118–123
    single posterior, 144–147
    two anterior, 132–139
  metal-ceramic
    anterior all-ceramic crowns with, 136–139
    single anterior implant-supported, 124–127
Cyan, 6, 11

D

D_{50} illuminant, 22–23, 23f–24f
D_{65} illuminant, 22–23, 24f
Dentin
  aging-related changes, 91f
  replacement of, 69, 72f–73f
Digital cameras, 83f, 83–84
Digital photography, 83f, 83–84
Digital Shade Guide, 98t–99t
Direct composite restorations
  anterior, 152–154
  case study of, 152–154
  dentin replacement, 69, 72f–73f
  enamel replacement, 69, 73f
  layering concepts for, 70, 71f–72f
  shade selection for, 72, 72f–74f

E

ΔE, 87–88
Easyshade, 98t–99t
Emission of light, 4–5
Emissive media, 10
Emotions, 40–41
Enamel replacement, 69, 72, 73f

F

Fabrication
  for conventional shade matching, 58f, 58–59
  for recommended shade-matching protocol, 110, 110f–111f
  for technological shade matching, 90
Fatigue, 40
Fluorescence, 45, 45f
Four-color processing, 12, 12f
Fovea, 21

G

Gray card, 16, 106, 108f, 112f
Green, 4t

H

"Hollywood" expectations, 54, 54f
Hue
  definition of, 15
  determination of, 61
  shade guides, 61
Hue contrast, 31t, 33–34, 34f

I

ikam, 98t–99t
Illuminants
  classification of, 21–22
  spectral data representation of, 24, 24f
  types of, 22f–26f, 22–26
Illumination
  description of, 20
  spectrophotometer, 85–86
Implant-supported metal-ceramic crown, 124–127
Indigo, 4t
International Commission on Illumination (CIE), 21–22
Interpretation
  for conventional shade matching, 58
  for recommended shade-matching protocol, 108, 108f–109f
  for technological shade systems, 89

Index

L
Layering, for direct composites, 70, 71f–72f
Light
  absorption of, 4–7
  emission of, 4–5
  intensity of, 21
  reflection of, 6, 6f–7f
  transmission of, 6, 6f
  wavelengths of, 2f
Light meter, 21f
Lighting
  color-corrected, 27, 28f
  conflicts in, 27
  incandescent, 28f
  metamerism, 28f, 28–30

M
Macular degeneration, 40
Magenta, 7, 11
Matching. *See* Shade matching.
Medications, 41, 41t
Metal-ceramic crown
  anterior all-ceramic crowns with, 136–139
  single anterior implant-supported, 124–127
Metameric pair, 29
Metamerism, 28f, 28–30
Meter
  color temperature, 27
  light, 21f
Miris shade guides, 71f–73f
Modern layering concept, 70, 71f
Munsell, Albert H., 14

N
Natural layering concept, 69
"Naturalist" expectations, 54, 55f
Nutrition, 40

O
Opacity, 52, 84f
Opalescence, 45–46, 46f
Oral contraceptives, 41
Orange, 4t, 34

P
Pigment colors, 12–14, 13t
Porcelain, 56
Posterior all-ceramic crowns, 144–147
Preoperative evaluations, 103
Primary colors
  additive, 10
  subtractive, 11, 11f
  types of, 13, 13f
Provisional restorations, 65f

R
Red, 4t, 13
Reflection of light, 6, 6f–7f
Reflective media, 10–11
Restorations
  direct composite. *See* Direct composite restorations.
  fabrication of, 58f, 58–59, 90, 110, 110f–111f
  placement of, 114, 114f–115f
Restorative materials
  fluorescence of, 45, 45f
  fracture toughness of, 44t
  opalescence of, 45, 46f
  selection of, 43–48
  translucency of, 44
Retina, 8, 8f
RGB color model, 10
RGB devices, 82–84
Rods, 8, 8f

S
Secondary colors, 13, 13f
Shade analysis. *See* Shade matching.
Shade guides
  Chromascop, 60
  description of, 59
  Miris, 71f–73f
  value-based, 61, 61f
  Vita Classical, 60, 64f
  Vitapan 3D-Master, 60–61, 64f
Shade map, 80
Shade matching
  aging effects on, 39
  color blindness effects on, 38–39
  conventional. *See* Conventional shade matching.
  D_{50} illuminants for, 24
  direct composites, 69–74
  emotions effect on, 40–41
  fatigue effects on, 40
  hue contrasts and, 35
  limitations of, 102, 102f
  preoperative patient evaluation for, 103
  recommended protocol for
    analysis, 104, 104f–105f
    communication, 106, 106f–107f
    fabrication, 110, 110f–111f
    interpretation, 108, 108f–109f
    placement, 114, 114f–115f
    verification, 112, 112f–113f
  technological. *See* Technological shade systems.
  time of day for, 27
Shade selection
  for direct composite restorations, 72, 72f–74f
  metamerism effects on, 30
Shade tabs, 56, 56f, 65f, 106
ShadeEye-NCC, 98t–99t
ShadeScan, 82, 82f, 98t–99t
ShadeVision, 98t–99t, 113f
Simultaneous contrast, 31–35
Spatial contrast, 31t, 37, 37f
Spectral curves, 24, 25f–26f
Spectral data
  definition of, 6
  illuminants represented as, 24, 24f
Spectrophotometers, 85f–86f, 85–86
SpectroShade, 79, 79f, 98t–99t, 105f, 113f
Spherical optics, 85
Spot measurement devices, 80–81, 91
Subtractive primary colors, 11, 11f

157

Index

Successive contrast, 31t, 37–38, 38f
Surface texture of teeth, 84f, 87, 90

T

Technological shade systems. *See also specific system.*
  colorimeters, 86–87
  description of, 78
  development of, 78–80
  digital cameras, 83f, 83–84
  early, 79
  future of, 97
  measurement systems, 80–81
  protocol for, 92–96, 93f–95f
  RGB devices, 82–84
  specifications for, 98t–99t
  spectrophotometers, 85f–86f, 85–86
  steps involved in
    analysis, 87–88
    communication, 89
    fabrication, 90
    interpretation, 89
    verification, 91
  summary of, 96–97
Teeth
  in adolescents, 90, 90f
  aging effects on, 90, 90f–91f
  bleached
    anterior ceramic laminate veneers matched to, 148–151
  color matching of, 53
  description of, 43–44, 44f, 47–48
  calcification of, 91f
  cleaning of, 72, 72f
  opacity of, 84f
  opalescence of, 45–46, 46f
  shade mapping of, 80
  surface texture of, 84f, 87, 90
  translucency of, 46, 46f, 64f, 84f, 90
Texture of teeth, 84f, 87
Transillumination, 45–46, 69f
Translucency
  definition of, 15–16, 16f
  of natural teeth, 46, 46f, 52, 53f, 64f, 84f, 90
  of restorative materials, 44
Transmission of light, 6, 6f
Transmissive media, 10–11
Trendy layering concept, 70, 71f
Tristimulus data, 9
Tyndall effect, 46

V

Value
  description of, 15, 44
  determination of, 61
  shade guides, 61
Value contrast, 31t, 32f–33f, 32–33
Veneers, anterior ceramic laminate, 128–131, 140–143
Verification
  for conventional shade matching, 59, 59f, 62
  for recommended shade-matching protocol, 112, 112f–113f
  for technological shade matching, 91
Violet, 4t
Visible light spectrum, 3
Vita Classical shade guide, 60, 64f
Vitapan 3D-Master shade guide, 60–61, 64f

W

Wavelengths
  absorption of, 7, 7f
  of colors, 3, 4t
  definition of, 3
  illustration of, 2f–3f
White light, 5

Y

Yellow, 4t, 11, 13, 34f